Transitions from Care to Independence

This important book focuses on the critical role of educational achievement for the well-being and success of vulnerable youth in adulthood. It is concerned with three interconnected issues: the support which is or should be afforded to youth ageing out of state care to enable them to fulfil their academic potential; the interdependence of social aspects of 'care' and educational attainment for children growing up in state care; and the conditions which are prerequisite for transition to fully autonomous adulthood, together with the implications of these for the state's responsibilities to care leavers.

These issues are addressed through a review of international literature based on the educational outcomes and life chances of youth graduating from state care, analysis of the findings of a three-year qualitative study following the educational transitions of young people and the use of theoretical frameworks to explore the complexities of children's experiences of the state care system. In doing so the book balances predominantly needs-based discourses with a children's rights perspective, focusing on competence rather than vulnerability and promoting the development of the skills needed for autonomous adulthood.

Transitions from Care to Independence should be considered essential reading for researchers, practitioners and policy-makers in the fields of education, childhood studies and adoption and fostering services. Additionally, the issues addressed are of wider relevance to youth transitions to adulthood. Youth ageing out of care provide a particularly insightful case study into the broader cohort of young people entering the workforce in an era of a globalised economy and austerity.

Jennifer Driscoll practised as a Family Law barrister for over a decade, specialising in child protection, before moving to King's in 2005, where she is Senior Lecturer in Child Studies. Her academic interests cover the protection and rights of vulnerable children, in particular child protection systems, the education of children and young people in and leaving state care, ethical issues arising from research with vulnerable children and young people and the implementation of the United Nations Convention on the Rights of the Child. Jenny is a member of the Board of Trustees of the British Association for the Study and Prevention of Child Abuse and Neglect (BASPCAN).

Routledge Advances in Social Work

https://www.routledge.com/Routledge-Advances-in-Social-Work/book-series/RASW

Transitions from Care to Independence

Supporting Young People Leaving State Care to Fulfil Their Potential

Jennifer Driscoll

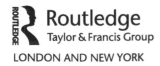
Routledge
Taylor & Francis Group

LONDON AND NEW YORK

First published 2018 by Routledge

2 Park Square, Milton Park, Abingdon, Oxfordshire OX14 4RN
52 Vanderbilt Avenue, New York, NY 10017

Routledge is an imprint of the Taylor & Francis Group, an informa business

First issued in paperback 2019

British Library Cataloguing-in-Publication Data
A catalogue record for this book is available from the British
Library

Library of Congress Cataloging-in-Publication Data
A catalog record for this book has been requested.

ISBN: 978-1-138-12293-2 (hbk)
ISBN: 978-0-367-43097-9 (pbk)

Typeset in Times New Roman
by codeMantra

Contents

List of tables

Acknowledgements

I feel privileged to have been granted some very moving insights into the lives of young people in state care through undertaking the study which inspired this book. Although they must remain anonymous, I thank all the young participants for their invaluable contribution, and particularly for the thoughtfulness and openness with which they responded to the intrusive questions of a stranger. I hope I have done justice to their personal testimonies, which I found both inspiring and motivating.

A study of this nature is not possible without significant support from professionals in schools and local authorities. I am very grateful to all of those who have taken time in their exceptionally busy working lives to participate and/or facilitate my research. That they have done so is both a testament to their professional dedication and evidence of the importance accorded to the topic by those working with young people in care. I am especially indebted to staff in the virtual schools at the local authorities I have named Stonycross and Riversmeet in the study and to the designated teachers at Woodhall and Fairfields.

My colleagues and friends have been enormously supportive and I have really valued the advice and expertise of colleagues in the School of Education, Communication & Society at King's College London, especially Professors Sharon Gewirtz and Meg Maguire. I would also particularly like to thank Professor Kathryn Hollingsworth and Dr Ann Lorek for their encouragement and insights.

Table of legislation/statutory instruments/ international instruments

Table of cases

Table of abbreviations

AAI	Adult Attachment Interview
AS/A2	Advanced Subsidiary/Advanced school level qualification usually taken by 16–18 year-olds (England and Wales)
ADHD	Attention Deficit Hyperactivity Disorder
ASFA	Adoption and Safe Families Act 1997 (US)
CAPTA	Child Abuse Prevention and Treatment Act 1974 (US)
CLET study	Care Leavers' Educational Transitions Study
DCSF	Department for Children, Schools and Families (England)
DfE	Department for Education (England)
ECHR	European Convention for the Protection of Human Rights and Fundamental Freedoms
FE	Further Education (UK) usually undertaken by young people aged 16–18
FFY	Federal fiscal year (US)
GAD	General Anxiety Disorder
GED	General Education Diploma (US)
GCSE	General Certificate of Secondary Education (England, Northern Ireland & Wales)
HE	Higher Education (UK) University/degree-level education
IOM	Institute of Medicine (US)
ICT	Information and Communication Technology
IRO	Independent Reviewing Officer (England & Wales)
NAIRO	National Association of Independent Reviewing Officers (England & Wales)
NCCMH	National Collaborating Centre for Mental Health (UK)
NEET	Not in education, employment or training
NIACE	National Institute of Adult Continuing Education (England and Wales)
NRC	National Research Council (US)
NS	National Statistics (UK)
OECD	Organisation for Economic Co-operation and Development
Ofsted	Office for Standards in Education, Children's Services and Skills (England)

PRU	Pupil Referral Unit
PTSD	Post-Traumatic Stress Disorder
RAD	Reactive Attachment Disorder
SDQ	Strengths and Difficulties Questionnaire
SEBD	Social, emotional and behavioural difficulties
SEU	Social Exclusion Unit (England)
SGO	Special Guardianship Order (England & Wales)
UASC	Unaccompanied Asylum-Seeking Children
UNCRC	United Nations Convention on the Rights for the Child
UNCoRC	United Nations Committee on the Rights of the Child
UNGA	United Nations General Assembly
USICH	United States Interagency Counil on Homelessness
VET	Vocational Education and Training
YiPPEE	Young People in Public Care: Pathways to Education in Europe project

1 Introduction

Introduction

Despite significant attention from policy-makers, outcomes for young people graduating from state care in Western countries have proven stubbornly resistant to improvement. As a consequence, such young adults are at significantly higher risk of poor life outcomes than their peers, including poverty, unemployment, homelessness, depression and anxiety, involvement in the criminal justice system and/or prostitution and those associated with young parenthood. This is the case in Europe and Scandinavia, as well as English-speaking Western jurisdictions, despite the variety of welfare and educational systems in different nations. In the drive to improve the life chances of youth ageing out of state care, two areas have been of particular focus: their educational attainment and the support available to youth as they transition out of care and into independent adulthood. Yet – perhaps because the majority have not entered further or higher education in the past – there has been little attention until recently to the education of youth in state care beyond the age of compulsory schooling, although rising proportions of young people entering tertiary education internationally reflect the importance of educational qualifications in advanced economies.

This book is concerned with three interconnected issues: first, the support which is or should be afforded to youth ageing out of care to enable them to fulfil their academic potential; second, the interdependence of social aspects of 'care' for children looked after by the state and their educational attainment; and third, the conditions which are pre-requisite for transition to fully autonomous adulthood and the implications of these for the state's responsibilities to care leavers. These issues are addressed through a review of the international literature base on the educational outcomes and life chances of youth graduating from state care; analysis of the findings of a three-year qualitative study following the educational transitions of English youth aged 15–18 (the Care Leavers' Educational Transitions (CLET) Study); and the use of four theoretical frameworks (attachment theory, Coleman's focal model of adolescence, resilience and foundational rights) to explore the complexities of children's experiences and needs before entering care, in care, and on leaving care. The use of a children's rights perspective is especially significant in an area in which a needs-based view has traditionally predominated and is employed here as a means by which to reconceptualise the role of the state as parent to children brought up in state care.

The issues addressed by the book are of wider relevance to youth transitions to adulthood. In the current globalised economy and as the Western world emerges from prolonged recession, developed nations attract an influx of immigrants willing and able to undertake jobs in which there is a skills deficit and/or unskilled and poorly remunerated jobs. The causes of youth unemployment and social exclusion in this context are complex and beyond the scope of this book, but while migrants may contribute significantly to the economy of host nations, youth who have grown up there but are unable to access skilled employment opportunities may be at increased risk of marginalisation and social exclusion in the globalised economy. Youth ageing out of care provide a particularly insightful case study into this broader cohort because they lack the support of families to cushion their transition to autonomous adulthood and rely entirely on the state to ensure that they reach their academic potential and are able to engage fully in society. I hope, therefore, that this book will contribute to the broader debate on how states can support their youth populations to maximise their potential to contribute to the economy and to society, a particular concern in both the United States of America (US) and the United Kingdom (UK), where there are wide inequalities in educational attainment.

The life chances of care leavers: an international perspective

My interest in the life circumstances of children brought up in the care of the state stems from my practice as a barrister in London, where I specialised in child protection. Two issues became prominent concerns in relation to the children who were the subject of the proceedings, almost none of whom I met, but whose lives were depicted through the evidence presented to the court. The first was the meagre support often offered to children and their families by children's social care authorities in the months and years prior to the decision to take proceedings to remove the children from the care of their parents. The high levels of harm suffered by children who were the subject of such proceedings and their consequent vulnerability underpins the second concern and this book, namely the long-term outcomes for young people who remain in care for the remainder of their childhood.

Removing children from the care of their parents is a draconian step. The appropriate balance between the protection of children and the rights of both children and parents to family life is an exceptionally difficult one to achieve (Fortin, 2009), but under English and international law, there is a strong emphasis on the rights of children and their parents to a family life together, and an assumption that in general, it is in a child's best interests to be brought up by his or her parents. Article 9 of the United Nations Convention on the Rights for the Child (UNCRC) (United Nations

General Assembly (UNGA), 1989) requires States Parties to ensure that children are not separated from their parents unless it is 'necessary for the best interests of the child' and cites 'abuse or neglect of the child by the parents' as an example of circumstances in which removal may be necessary. Although the UNCRC has been directly incorporated into national law in relatively few states and lacks effective mechanisms for implementation of its provisions, all countries except for the US have ratified the Convention.

The state can only justify taking over the parental role in relation to children if it is also able to provide 'better' parenting and improved outcomes in adulthood than would have been the case if the child had remained in the care of his or her parents. As a result of their pre-care experiences, these children require high standards of parenting if they are to recover from the experiences of their earlier years and reach their potential in adulthood. Under article 20 of the UNCRC (1989), a 'child temporarily or permanently deprived of his or her family environment, or in whose best interests cannot be allowed to remain in that environment, shall be entitled to special protection and assistance provided by the state'. It is, however, difficult if not impossible to assess the extent to which state care can or does improve the lives of the children entrusted to it. As Cutuli et al. (2016) note, inadequacies in the data available limit our understanding of long-term outcomes for this group of children. Currently there are limited available data on the outcomes for care leavers in much of the world, including Africa, China, India, South America (Pinkerton, 2011) and most post-communist countries (Stein, 2014). However, the available evidence in developed countries provides considerable cause for concern, with reviews suggesting care fails to improve children's prospects and in some cases may make them worse (Goemans et al., 2015; Maclean et al., 2016). In English-speaking nations, Lonne et al. (2009) have described care leavers' adult outcomes as 'deplorable' (173), a view supported in England by Stein (2006b) and Jackson (2007) and in the US by numerous studies (see Bender et al., 2015, for a summary).

Poor outcomes in adulthood are inextricably linked to the difficulties experienced by care leavers in obtaining adequate and lasting employment (see Courtney et al., 2007; Jackson and Cameron, 2010), which in turn are consequent upon the generally poor educational attainment of this cohort. Although English research has elucidated factors associated with the high achievement of children in care (Jackson et al., 2005; Chase et al., 2006), a systematic review of 28 studies from Australia, Canada, the UK and the US (O'Higgins et al., 2015) concluded that as a cohort, children in care perform less well educationally than their peers in relation to attainment, attendance and exclusion. This correlation is partly explained by children's experiences before entering into care, and the attainment gap is reduced once individual characteristics of the child (including ethnicity, gender and Special Educational Needs) are accounted for (O'Higgins et al., 2015). The review concluded that although there was little evidence to suggest that care impacts negatively on children's educational outcomes, neither does it appear to enhance them.

More generally, there is a dearth of research on young people's experiences of transitioning out of care (McCoy et al., 2008, in the US). Wade and Munro (2008) conclude that understanding of the challenges facing young people leaving care remains greater than that of effective transitions to support their transition to independence. Currently only six per cent of English care leavers enter higher education by the age of 19 (DfE/NS, 2013), roughly the same proportion as in Denmark and Sweden (Jackson and Cameron, 2011). Perhaps as a consequence, the educational participation and attainment of care leavers and especially their experience of educational transitions are under-researched in the European context (Höjer et al., 2008; Jackson and Cameron, 2010; Bluff et al., 2012), a factor which motivated the study that is the focus of this book. This area of enquiry is important not only in its own right but also by reason of the wider lessons that can be learnt from the experiences of this population and applied to other groups of young people.

The wider policy implications of outcomes for children from state care

Children in the care of the state comprise a relatively small cohort at one end of a continuum of children for whom there are concerns about their welfare or safety. In reality, children do not fall neatly into categories of need and risk, but for legal and administrative purposes they must be classified according to the extent to which state intervention into their families' lives is deemed to be justified. To use the US as an example, in the federal fiscal year (FFY) 2013, around 3.5 million referrals were made to child protection agencies, concerning about 6.4 million children (U.S. Department of Health and Human Services, Administration for Children and Families, Administration on Children, Youth and Families, Children's Bureau, 2015). 2.1 million of those referrals led to further action, with 3.2 million children the subject of investigation or alternative response and nearly 1.3 million receiving post-response services from a child protection agency: roughly one-third of the latter were removed from home. 679,000 children were identified as victims of maltreatment (9.1 per thousand children in the population), including an estimated 1,520 children who had died (just over two per thousand children).

These figures are a reflection of the enormous increase in referrals to children's social care services experienced by developed nations in the last 30 to 40 years (Lonne et al., 2009), attributable to a large extent to greater professional awareness and the development of child protection policies and systems (Gardner and Brandon, 2008). Nonetheless, maltreatment remains under-reported in high-income countries (Gilbert et al., 2009a). The upshot of these factors combined is that many children living in circumstances which may compromise their welfare or development (such as in the care of adults who misuse drugs or alcohol or have mental health difficulties or in households where there is intimate partner violence) remain unknown to social care services. Concurrently, children's social care services, investment in which has not kept pace with the responsiveness of professionals in universal services, have come under increased resourcing pressures, resulting in deficiencies in organisational capacity and high thresholds for state intervention (see e.g. Ofsted, 2008; IOM and NRC, 2014).

Many children who are not in state care live 'on the edges' of the child protection system in circumstances in which the professionals to whom they are known are concerned for their welfare but have limited options at their disposal by which to assist them. It is also important to note the transitory nature of many children's encounters with the care system. English figures, for example, show that less than half of the children in care at any time in the year ending 31st March 2016 had been in care continuously for at least 12 months (DfE/NS, 2016a).

So what are the implications of these blurred boundaries of risk and intervention for child protection and education policy? Young people with poor outcomes in adulthood who do not come from a care background may nonetheless have experienced remarkably similar childhood adversities to care leavers, including poverty, maltreatment and family conflict. In a study of homeless youth, Bender et al. (2015) found 'surprisingly few differences' (228) between the living contexts and needs of those from a foster care background and those without, attributed to the common risk factors in both groups. The authors identified the important differences between the groups as being of degree: the foster youth had suffered greater abuse and neglect than their peers on the streets, and they had been homeless for longer. In the UK the term 'safeguarding' has been adopted to reflect the concept of a continuum of need and risk and the importance of focusing not merely on protecting children whose cases meet the legal 'threshold' for removal from care, but also on the promotion of child welfare and early intervention to safeguard children from further harm. In relation to educational attainment and outcomes in early adulthood, the inference to be drawn from the notion of a continuum of harm is that interventions or ways of working that are successful in improving the life chances of those children who have suffered the most harmful childhood experiences have much wider potential to benefit the vast numbers of children who are living in chaotic or risky home circumstances.

The English policy context

The English policy context is a useful one for the purposes of international comparison and analysis because research in this area is of longer standing than in most other developed nations, thanks to the seminal work of Sonia Jackson in the late 1980s, and there has been sustained policy attention to children in state care as a distinct group. Following the introduction of provisions for the review of 'looked after' children's welfare in the Children Act 1989, political attention to the fate of this group of children increased (Jackson, 2013a), and they came to the fore in policy under New Labour[1] (Smith, 2009) as part of wider attempts to tackle social exclusion (Social Exclusion Unit, 2003). Since the turn of the century, there has been considerable legislative and policy activity aimed at improving the life chances of children who have experienced state care, including through the Children (Leaving Care) Act 2000, Children Act 2004, Children and Young Persons Act 2008, the Children and Families Act 2014 and the Children and Social Work Act 2017. At the start of the CLET study, the role of a 'designated teacher for looked-after children' had recently been made statutory through section 20 of the Children and Young Persons Act 2008, while the post of 'virtual school head for looked-after children', now a statutory requirement pursuant to section 98 of the Children and Families Act 2014, had been the subject of a recent pilot.

The past few years have produced some evidence that the political initiatives of the last 15 to 20 years have begun to take effect, including a slight narrowing of the attainment gap between children in care and their peers at age 16, when children take GCSE (General Certificate of Secondary Education) examinations. Yet policies designed to improve the educational attainment of children in care have been slow to make any measureable impact (Jackson, 2010), and the gap between the educational achievement of this cohort and their peers remains large: in 2015, 14 per cent of children in care achieved the government benchmark of five GCSEs at A*-C including mathematics and English, compared with 53 per cent of the general population (DfE/NS, 2016b). However, recent research in England (Sebba et al., 2015) concludes that children who experience relatively longer stays in care perform better than those 'in need' (a group of children identified as being in need of social care services pursuant to statutory definitions but who remain in the care of their birth families: they can roughly be considered equivalent to the 'in-home' care cohorts in international studies).

This book starts from the premise that the educational experiences and attainment of children in state care can be understood only in the wider context of their lives and care (Jackson, 2013a). The circumstances leading to their entry into care combined with their unique status as the children of the state (referred to as the 'corporate parent' in England) affect all aspects of their lives at home and in school. English policy and practice have moved broadly from a position of low professional expectations of children's achievement in school in deference to their care needs (Jackson, 2010) to one which has tended to regard education as a panacea for all social ills and consequently as a primary policy focus for a range of groups of disadvantaged children. Through the CLET study, I have attempted to reconcile these opposing policy stances by examining them for the advancement of children's educational achievement in the context of theoretical frameworks which explain the unique challenges faced by children in care and by foregrounding the perspectives of young people ageing out of care.

The care leavers' educational transitions study

The majority of the existing research on the education of children in care focuses on children of compulsory school age, although researchers in England have followed some of the small proportion of care leavers entering higher education through their degree courses (Jackson et al., 2003, 2005; Ajayi and Quigley, 2006). Less attention has been paid to whether, and if so how, care leavers reaching the statutory school-leaving age with disappointing qualifications can be supported to make up any educational deficit. Although the statutory school-leaving age remained 16 at the time of the study (2011–13), legislation which requires young people to continue to participate in education or training until the age of 18 was being introduced (Education and Skills Act 2008, Part 1 and Education Act 2011, section 74). Consideration of the effect of recent policy initiatives to encourage greater participation by care leavers in further and higher education was therefore particularly timely.

The overarching aim of the study was to explore how young people in care experience educational transitions in upper secondary school and how these transitions might best be supported. This is a critical time in young people's lives because they are required to make decisions which are likely to influence their future career trajectories and life chances to a significant degree. Although there is now a significant body of English research on the education of children in care, the dearth of research evidence in relation to the role of designated teachers (senior members of school staff responsible for the education of this group of children) reflects a wider lack of research in relation to the import of *schools* in the lives of this group (Berridge et al., 2008). This is a significant gap, given that teachers are the adults most commonly cited as being supportive of their education by children in care (Harker et al., 2004).

The main objectives of the study were:

1 To explore the key barriers to academic progress for older school children ageing out of care and how they experience and navigate these barriers;
2 To consider the interdependence of young people's experiences in and before entering care and their educational outcomes in order better to understand the most effective means by which young people may be supported through and in education;
3 To assess the effectiveness of educational initiatives intended to promote the engagement and progress of care leavers in education; and
4 To identify how young people transitioning out of care might best be supported to fulfil their educational potential.

Children ageing out of care in England are likely also to experience transitions in other areas of their lives during this period, compounded for many by late entrance into care. Accordingly, I chose to undertake a longitudinal study to capture young people's experiences of these multiple transitions and the effect of decisions that they made on their life in very early adulthood. A longitudinal design is relatively rare in research with children in care and care leavers, probably because the transient nature of many children's encounters with the care system and the instability of their lives in care render such projects challenging and resource-intensive: this is a notoriously 'hard-to-reach' group. 21 young people aged 15–16 were recruited in the first year of the study with the aim of interviewing them each year over a three-year period. As a result of attrition during the study, 45 interviews with young people were undertaken in total. In addition, interviews were conducted with 12 of the designated teachers or safeguarding officers in the young people's schools and colleges and five professionals from local government 'virtual schools' which hold responsibility for the education of all children in care in their local authority area, making a total of 65 interviews in the study overall. A more detailed account of the methodology and methodological issues is set out in Appendix 1, including tables showing the characteristics of participants and the pattern of interviews with young people.

The central tenet underpinning the theoretical perspectives and methodological choices selected for the study is a commitment to children's rights, which led me to focus my attention on the experiences and views of care leavers themselves. While children in the UK have been accorded protection rights on the basis of their developmental immaturity and vulnerability since at least the 19th century, the notion that children should enjoy a comparable range of rights to those of adults, including some degree of autonomy, is still a relatively new one and remains contested, although it has gained significant momentum from the implementation of the UNCRC (UNGA, 1989; Fortin, 2009). The UNCRC includes as one of its core principles a child's right to participate in decisions affecting him or her, which is set out in article 12. Article 12 performs an important role in facilitating the child's acquisition of the necessary competencies to prepare him or her for autonomous adulthood, through recognition of the significance of children's social experiences in developing their decision-making capacities.

This principle may be regarded as of particular significance to care leavers. Research involving young people engages their participation rights under the UNCRC, an especially meaningful exercise in relation to marginalised groups (Wigfall and Cameron, 2006). Winter concluded in 2006 that 'the detailed accounts of looked-after children themselves' are missing from the literature (Winter, 2006: 55), complaining that the approach adopted in most research

> does not easily accommodate a view of looked-after children as active, skilled and competent agents in social processes and therefore does not fully engage with their participation rights.

> (58)

Rather, she contended, research tends to be founded on a view of children as recipients of a service, the outcomes of which are defined by adult values. Such an approach is likely to compound the powerlessness of children in care, whose experience of corporate parenting often centres on being on the receiving end of decisions over which they have no influence (Leeson, 2007).

Incongruently however, care leavers are generally expected to achieve independence earlier than their peers (Stein, 2006a), rendering attention to their participation rights of particular importance. The participants in this study were aged 15 to 18, a life stage at which young people are becoming increasingly autonomous and during which they make a number of important decisions which may materially affect their outcomes in adult life. While the fact that children and adults often have different perspectives does not imply that either view is 'right' or 'wrong' (Holland, 2009: 232), the perspectives of young people are the driving force behind their decisions and, therefore, of primary significance. Moreover, care leavers often have a strong sense of self-reliance (Cameron, 2007) and a particular sense of identity arising from their fractured experience of family life, which renders research into their own perspectives of particular value, as Samuels and Pryce (2008) attest in relation to fostered children in the US. The diversity of experiences of children in care combined with the commonalities in their pre-care experiences across different countries and the range of social care systems internationally suggests that the evidence of care leavers themselves is likely to be of greatest value in understanding their pathways from care to independence.

Theoretical perspectives

There has generally been limited attention to the use of theoretical frameworks to develop understanding of the experiences of care leavers (Stein, 2006b; Lee and Berrick, 2014), and this study provided an opportunity to explore the potential of a number of theoretical models to afford greater insight into the challenges facing young people. Stein (2006b) has proposed attention to attachment theory, Coleman's focal model of adolescence (Coleman, 1974) and resilience as potentially fruitful areas of enquiry. These three conceptual frameworks are all utilized in the following chapters to illuminate children's experiences in and leaving care, but insights from each are interrogated from the perspective of children's rights.

Attachment theory (Bowlby, 1969) is an evolutionary theory that posits that infants seek proximity to their primary caregiver(s) (or 'attachment figure') in the face of threat (Prior and Glaser, 2006). It is of particular pertinence to children in state care because of their experiences of maltreatment, removal from their parents and, often, multiple changes of placement. Although there is much controversy over the use of attachment theory and associated therapies with children in care (Osuwu-Bempah, 2010), it remains the most appropriate lens through which to view the complex feelings young people have towards their birth and foster families and has implications for their ability to build relationships in adulthood.

The concept of resilience, a term used to signify positive adaptation in the face of significant adverse experiences (Luthar and Cicchetti, 2000), has perhaps attracted the most interest from researchers working with care leavers. Resilience theory provides a flexible framework through which to incorporate consideration of the range of protective and risk factors that impact on the lives of children in care and facilitates a strengths-based perspective which acknowledges children's agency. It is particularly well suited to this study because good educational experiences are associated with resilient adaptation (Masten et al., 1990; Luthar and Cicchetti, 2000). In the pilot study for this project, self-reliance (a quality which may be a source of resilience) was a key theme arising from interviews with care leavers. Cameron has identified two dimensions to self-reliance: 'having confidence in oneself to manage one's own affairs; and preferring not to have help' (2007: 39). Self-reliance is generally a positive attribute but may operate as a barrier to accessing professional support (Cameron, 2007), an important consideration in this study. Used in combination, attachment theory and the concept of self-reliance can shed light on the deep-rooted mistrust of key adults in their lives so often exhibited by care leavers.

The longitudinal design of the study enabled me to consider the potential insights offered by Coleman's focal model of adolescence, which suggests that young people actively manage the developmental tasks of adolescence in a sequential manner. The focal model provides insight into the particular challenges faced by care leavers, who are likely to encounter multiple transitions as they age out of care. Stein has described care leavers in Europe as experiencing 'accelerated and compressed' transitions to adulthood, whilst the transition from care to independence is 'abrupt and extended' in post-communist countries (Stein, 2006a: 274; 2014: 35). The focal model helps to explain why care leavers may struggle to focus on making up any educational deficits with which they have entered care, while often concurrently facing upheaval in their personal lives, at a time when they are also tackling the developmental tasks of adolescence and may still be subject to significant emotional trauma.

Consequently, many care leavers are ill-equipped for independence in the modern world when they attain the age of legal majority, as indeed are many of their peers who have not been in care. Arguably, the welfare-based paradigm in which children in state care are conceptualised as vulnerable and treated as the objects of professional concern may serve to exacerbate the challenges facing young people required to achieve independence earlier than their peers. Research evidence from England suggests that children in care continue to feel excluded from many of the key decisions affecting them (Cameron, 2007; Leeson, 2007; Morgan, 2014). A rights-based approach which recognises young people's evolving capacities and their claim to promotion of their developing autonomy can help to emphasise children's claims to be fully involved in decisions affecting them and to focus on their competence rather than their vulnerability, promoting the development of the skills needed for autonomous adulthood.

A rights-based discourse has become increasingly dominant internationally since the near-universal ratification of the UNCRC (UNGA, 1989), although children's claims to autonomy rights still attract less attention than their rights to care and protection. The implications of respect for children's autonomy rights in a study of this nature are three-fold. First, children's voices remain marginalised in policy and practice, yet article 12 of the UNCRC requires that states 'assure to the child who is capable of forming his or her own views the right to express those views freely in all matters affecting the child, the views of the child being given due weight in accordance with the age and maturity of the child'. This provision relates not only to matters pertaining to children's individual experiences but also to the provision of services and the development of policies affecting groups of children (United Nations Committee on the Rights of the Child, 2009: 5). For this reason, I chose to foreground the views of young people in the study. Second, on the cusp of adulthood, young people's own perspectives are most significant in understanding the driving forces behind the decisions that they make about their futures. Third, understanding how care leavers can make a successful transition to adulthood entails consideration of the conditions required for exercise of autonomy in independent adulthood. In relation to this latter point, there has been some criticism that rights-based analyses tend to pay inadequate attention to the primacy of relationships in social work, exacerbating the instrumentalist approach to the entitlements of young people to state resources exhibited by legislative solutions (Smith, 2009). Recent developments in the theorisation of children's rights have, however, addressed this deficit by incorporating considerations of relational capabilities developed by Nussbaum (2003) into understandings of the development of autonomy (Hollingsworth, 2013b). In this book I draw on Hollingsworth's theory of foundational rights, which incorporates consideration of relational autonomy, in order to analyse the full basis of children's rights to ongoing state support beyond the age of legal majority.

The structure of the book

I draw together the international literature on the educational outcomes and life chances of youth graduating from state care to focus attention on the critical role of educational achievement in the well-being and success of vulnerable youth in adulthood in this book. But I also explore the interdependence of care and education and the implications of that relationship for the concept of the state as 'corporate parent', as well as for social care and education systems and policy and practice in relation to children in state care. I evaluate the way in which social attitudes and public policy in relation to vulnerable youth may serve to perpetuate their marginalisation through analysis of the meaning and achievement of full equality of educational opportunity. Finally, I address the dearth of theoretical work in this area and employ a children's rights analysis to reconsider the responsibilities of the state towards youth in its direct care.

Chapter 2 provides a brief account of the social and political drivers of social policy and child welfare/protection systems and trends in alternative care provision in Western countries, together with a summary of the potential contribution of a social pedagogic approach to the care of maltreated children. Insights from these sections are used to address the complexity in evaluating alternative care regimes and to highlight the implications for child welfare of alternative care as a measure of last resort. To inform analysis of the challenges facing children ageing out of state care, the developmental tasks of adolescence are explored through the lens of Coleman's focal model of adolescence. Care leavers' transitions to adulthood are compared with those of their peers in an era of 'emerging adulthood', in which young people remain dependent on their families for longer. Recent developments in state support for care leavers in recognition of this trend are set out. In conclusion, the responsibilities owed by the state to children for whom it has taken on a parenting role are conceptualised through a children's rights perspective, using Hollingsworth's theory of foundational rights.

The first of two chapters concerned with children's experiences of the care system, Chapter 3 considers the impact of maltreatment on child development and welfare and uses insights from attachment theory to understand their experiences and needs. The association between maltreatment and attachment issues is considered, together with the implications of attachment behaviours for the care of maltreated children. These accounts from the literature provide a context for examining the empirical data on the personal histories of the young participants in the CLET study, including their experiences of loss, bereavement and rejection, and their relationships with birth family members. Next, the literature on placement stability is considered as a prelude to analysis of study participants' accounts of their lives in care, with particular attention to placement disruption and relationships with carers. The final section considers the effect of young people's personal experiences before entering care and in care on their educational continuity and engagement.

Chapter 4 explores the experience of 'being in care' and 'corporate parenting' and the impact on young people's daily lives from the perspectives of both young people and professionals, including issues of stigma and trust, surveillance and bureaucracy, and impersonal and transient relationships with social workers. The cumulative effect of these experiences is analysed through the concept of self-reliance, widely regarded as an aspect of resilience. The notion of resilient adaptation and insights from the 'coping' literature are employed in order to consider the ways in which the resilience of children in care and care leavers might best be promoted. In the final section, the congruities between the theoretical lenses of attachment, resilience, the focal model and foundational rights are reviewed to draw together findings on the importance of relational aspects of the lives of young people ageing out of the care system.

Chapter 5 addresses the importance of educational attainment for adult well-being, including self-worth, autonomy and 'success', and the significance of education for social mobility and in enhancing the prospects of marginalised or disadvantaged groups of youth. Recent changes in policy to meet the skills needs of developed economies, including raising the age of compulsory education or training and extension of tertiary education to a larger proportion of the population, are considered. The young CLET study participants' views on the importance of education are discussed, and the international literature on the educational achievement of children in state care in relation to their peers, including entry to further (16–18) and higher (tertiary) education, is reviewed. Adult outcomes for graduates of care 'systems' internationally are compared, including in relation to socio-economic and employment status, mental and physical health, homelessness and involvement in the criminal justice system.

Initiatives to support the education of children in care and care leavers are briefly reviewed in Chapter 6, with particular attention to the introduction of 'designated teachers' in educational settings and 'virtual school heads' at local government level in England. Detailed discussion of the insights gained from the CLET study on supporting children in school and in their post-16 educational pathways is provided, including designated teachers' and young people's conceptualisation of 'success', young people's aspirations and their commitment to educational achievement, the role of carers in supporting young people's educational progress and the choices and challenges faced by young people in their post-16 pathways. Evidence of a significant shift in professional attitudes to children's attainment is presented, together with consideration of the extent to which young people were able to realise their aspirations and/or reach their academic potential in qualifications taken at 16 and developments in supporting young people in their education beyond 16.

The polarisation of participants' trajectories over the three years of the study is considered in relation to key theoretical and policy perspectives in Chapter 7. Attachment theory and Coleman's focal model of adolescence are used to explore the implications of young people's experiences of transitions in multiple domains of their lives as they graduate from state care to independence. Participants' preoccupation with relationships with their birth family members and the reassessment of their relationships with carers as they age out of care are discussed. Stein's categorisation of care leavers based on resilient adaptation is employed to summarise the effect of risk and protective factors in young people's lives and the role of self-reliance in their choices and outcomes to date. The motivation for and implications of some young people's active choices to move to live independently are addressed in order to understand young people's pathways to the situations they found themselves in at the end of the study and the very diverse futures that they appeared to be facing.

Young people's care outcomes are evaluated in Chapter 8 using insights from Hollingsworth's concept of foundational rights, which incorporates consideration not only of concrete capabilities such as educational attainment but also of relational aspects of autonomy. The concept is used to elucidate the duties corporate parents should owe to the children in their care, facilitated through an analysis of what young people need in order to be prepared to exercise genuine or 'full' autonomy in adulthood. The tendency for recent policy and practice to privilege more academically successful young people is considered through Goldson's notion of the '"deserving" – "underserving" schism', together with the challenges inherent in the corporate parenting model in meeting the individual needs of children in care. The role of designated teachers and virtual school heads in improving the educational and life outcomes for care leavers is evaluated, and the extent to which the principles of social pedagogy have potential to promote a more holistic and relationship-based approach to work with children in care and care leavers is discussed.

The final chapter reviews the key findings of the CLET study and evaluates the study's contribution to the empirical research literature. The significance of insights from the findings for theoretical framings of the state's responsibilities to the children for whom it has assumed responsibility are considered, particularly as young people approach and attain legal adulthood. Fruitful directions for further research in this area are suggested. The implications of the findings in the international context for policy and practice affecting this small cohort of disadvantaged young people who have a particular claim on the state to safeguard and promote their welfare are briefly summarised.

Note

1 The name given to the Centre Left government in power under Prime Ministers Tony Blair and Gordon Brown (1997–2010) which combined free market economy thinking with principles of social justice, an approach known as the 'third way'.

2 Alternative care

The systems

The politics of care: social context, social policy and social care

The roots of state systems for children's social care in Western nations lie in charitable and philanthropic work originally undertaken by religious and voluntary groups (Hessle, 2013). In the late 19th-century 'child rescue' movements sprang up, such as the New York Society for the Prevention of Cruelty to Children, formed in 1874. Campaigns for acceptance of state responsibility led to the birth of modern child welfare systems across Europe, the US and Scandinavia (Wolff et al., 2011; Hessle, 2013; Pösö et al., 2014). Broadly, in English-speaking countries, the premise of state non-intervention in family life led to the development of child protection (or child safety) oriented systems designed to allow intervention only in situations evaluated to be high-risk. In mainland Europe and Scandinavia, the family welfare (or child and family welfare) model saw provision of broad state services for the support of families, of which intervention for the protection of children is just one aspect (see Katz and Hetherington, 2006; Healy and Oltedal, 2010; Gilbert et al. 2011; Hessle, 2013) for evaluations as to these categorisations by countries). This dichotomous classification is, however, a simplistic one. Many modern child protection systems lie on a continuum between these two positions, while systems vary over time in response to the political, social and cultural climate. Hessle (2013) suggests that evaluation of national child welfare systems requires consideration of three interdependent dimensions: family policy in the context of wider social welfare policy, socio-cultural context and child welfare policy in relation to the welfare-protection continuum described above.

Social policy systems

Esping-Andersen (1990) developed a three-fold typology of social policy systems. In the liberal model, which he originally identified in the US, Canada and Australia, with approximations in Denmark, Sweden and the UK, the state is minimized in favour of market forces and the focus is on risk reduction rather than welfare promotion (Healy and Oltedal, 2010), tending to result in privatisation of services and the perpetuation of unequal life chances (Scruggs and Allan, 2008). In practice, this has translated into fewer resources being invested in preventative work in English-speaking countries than in European and Nordic countries (Katz and Hetherington, 2006). Lonne et al. (2009) attribute what they regard as systemic failures in child protection systems in Anglophone countries at least in part to the influence of neoliberal and market-oriented policies, arguing that a focus on individual responsibility fails to accord sufficient significance to structural factors such as poverty and adopts a punitive response to parental inadequacies. The corporativist or conservative model, assigned by Esping-Andersen originally to Austria, France, Germany and Italy, although featuring significant state investment in social welfare (Scruggs and Allan, 2008), tends to be paternalistic and reinforce traditional family structures (Esping-Andersen, 1990). Service delivery is likely to rely on voluntary or religious organisations (Katz and Hetherington, 2006), which may result in a lack of established common standards (Spratt et al., 2015, in relation to Germany). The social democratic welfare model, seen in Norway and Sweden, and to an extent in Denmark and Finland (Esping-Andersen, 1990), exhibits a willingness to accept high levels of investment in social services in the interests of equality of opportunity. These countries are 'statist' in the concentration of service delivery through state institutions, but in recent years the governments of Nordic countries such as Norway have been influenced by aspects of neoliberal policy (Healy and Oltedal, 2010).

Socio-cultural context

The principle that family life is the preferred environment for the upbringing of children has been universally endorsed through the UN *Guidelines for the Alternative Care of Children* (UNGA, 2010) (IIA3), which state that removal of the child from familial care should be 'a measure of last resort' and last for 'the shortest possible duration' (IIB14). Removal of a child from parents' care is a breach of the right of children and parents to family life under article 8(1) of the European Convention for the Protection of Human Rights and Fundamental Freedoms (ECHR). European Court of Human Rights jurisprudence stresses that the level of state intervention in family life must be a proportionate response to the circumstances (*Haase* v *Germany*, 2004) and that removal from parents should be regarded as a temporary measure (*Johansen* v *Norway*, 1996). Nordic countries adhere particularly strongly to this principle: in-home services must be demonstrated to have been ineffective before placements out of the home will be countenanced (Pösö et al., 2014). In Sweden, whether children are removed under voluntary agreement or compulsory state intervention, the placement aim is rehabilitation home (Khoo and Skoog, 2014).

In English law, before ordering the removal of a child from his or her parents the court must be satisfied that the child is 'suffering or likely to suffer significant harm' (Children Act 1989 section 31(2)). A similarly high bar is set in the US under the Child Abuse Prevention and Treatment Act 1974 (CAPTA) and the Adoption and Safe Families Act 1997 (ASFA), which set strict time limits for the making of decisions either to return children in care to their parents or terminate parental rights in preparation for adoption, although reunification attempts may be dispensed with in cases of sexual abuse and prolonged physical abuse (Myers, 2008). As a consequence, children entering state care are likely to have experienced a lengthy period of maltreatment or inadequate parenting and have high levels of need across all domains of their lives, but they may face further instability through moving in and out of care.

Western family welfare services share a pattern of disproportionate representation of certain groups. Despite widespread efforts to address discrimination, children from foreign countries (Hessle, 2013), indigenous children in Australia, Canada, New Zealand and the US (Lonne et al., 2009) and ethnic minority children remain over-represented in care systems and in alternative care placements. Although the reasons for this pattern persisting are unclear (Owen and Statham, 2009), it is widely attributed to culturally-biased assumptions as to appropriate parenting practices, coupled with the likelihood that ethnic minority or indigenous families are socioeconomically disadvantaged compared with the general population.

A significant difference between nations lies in the status accorded to care work and work with children. In many jurisdictions, child protection remains low-status work, reflecting both the lack of prestige accorded to the nature of the work and the low social status of families coming into contact with child protection services (Healy and Oltedal, 2010). The highly regulated and overstretched services in English-speaking countries are associated with high levels of staff turnover and problems in recruitment as well as poor training and supervision (Munro, 2011; Lonne et al., 2013). The social democratic welfare state is in principle more sympathetic to demands for investment in children, both in the interests of social equality and in pursuit of high levels of employment to sustain the welfare state: Healy and Oltedal (2010) found the Norwegian workforce to be more stable than that in Queensland, Australia. Work with children is also of higher status in continental European countries than in the English-speaking world, and a contributing factor in that context is the development of social pedagogy practice. Nonetheless, recruitment and retention of high-quality foster carers is a universal issue, identified in countries including Australia, France, Japan, Sweden, the UK and the US (Colton et al., 2008; Norgate, 2012; Randle et al., 2016).

The welfare-protection continuum

It is challenging to assess the success of different child protection systems, not only as a result of hybridisation over time but also because of the lack of directly comparable data and variations in the context and structure of the different systems (Katz and Hetherington, 2006), even setting aside questions about what constitutes 'success' in relation to the work of child protection systems. Nonetheless, significant differences are evident in patterns of state intervention in the family, and some of the advantages and disadvantages of different models have been identified.

Contact with family welfare-oriented systems is less likely to be perceived as stigmatising by parents, providing greater capacity for constructive relationships between professionals and parents (Katz and Hetherington, 2006). Thresholds for state intervention or support are likely to be higher in child protection systems: in Pecora et al.'s (2006) US study of 659 young adult family foster care alumni, 93 per cent suffered maltreatment inflicted by their birth family. In England, roughly 0.6 per cent of the child population is in care at any one time (DfE/NS, 2016a). In some countries, more than double that proportion of children are placed in state care: in Finland the figure is around 1.2 per cent (Pösö et al., 2014). Emphasis on family support, a reluctance to resort to compulsory intervention and less stigma surrounding growing up in care result in most children being placed into care through voluntary arrangements in Scandinavian countries such as Finland (Pösö et al., 2014). In contrast, only 27 per cent of children in care in England are voluntarily accommodated (DfE/NS, 2016).

The family welfare system is not necessarily as successful as might be expected, however. The presumption that services will work in partnership with parents to support the integrity of the family unit may lead to children suffering maltreatment over a longer period (Pösö et al., 2014). Adolescents make up a particularly large proportion of the care population in Nordic countries (Socialstyrelsen, 2011, cited in Khoo et al., 2012; Pösö et al., 2014). These figures are affected by the fact that juvenile delinquency and criminal conduct are dealt with through the welfare system in Nordic countries. Nonetheless, in a review of studies comparing outcomes for children from the child protection system with those in the general population, Poso et al. (2014) conclude that in Denmark, Norway and Finland, care leavers experience poorer health, educational outcomes and employment prospects. These youth struggle to develop secure relationships and are at greater risk of premature death and suicide compared with their peers. The studies question the assumption that the arrangements in Nordic states are superior to those elsewhere, pointing out that the evidence base for supportive in-home services remains scanty.

Universally, increased professional awareness and identification coupled with a widening of the scope of child-rearing practices regarded as harmful have resulted in high levels of referral, arguably exacerbated by mandatory reporting requirements in many nations. Child protection systems have become overwhelmed with tasks of filtering and risk assessment, while family welfare systems have come under strain from recessionary pressures (Lonne et al., 2009; Hessle, 2013; Petersen et al., 2014). However, concurrently, there has been heightened awareness of the long-term economic costs of maltreatment and the development of a view which regards children as a social investment (Spratt et al., 2015), leading to a shift by child protection-oriented systems towards greater emphasis on prevention and early intervention (e.g. valentine and Katz, 2015, in Australia). This shift is evident in England, where the child protection system might be described as the result of a 'hands-off' government approach modified by a reactive stance to specific events in the national context (see e.g. Munro, 2011).

The features of child protection systems described above affect not just the age and experiences of children entering care and the length of time they are likely to spend there, but also their experiences while in care and their life outcomes. Lonne et al. (2009) describe systems in English-speaking nations as characterised by surveillance, 'dominated by forensic investigation and yet unable to provide effective help to the vulnerable and those in need, *particularly children in care*' (page 175, my emphasis). The next section briefly sets out alternative care arrangements in Western nations and describes the European social pedagogy model, which offers a distinctive perspective on the care of maltreated children.

Alternative care regimes: the international picture

The decades following the Second World War saw a shift in Western nations from the use of large institutional children's homes to family-based care. This phenomenon reflected experiences of the widespread evacuation of children from their families during the War, the publication of Bowlby's work *Child Care and the Growth of Love* in 1953 (Frost & Stein, 1989) and recognition of the right to family life. In Germany, youth revolts ('Heimkampagnen' or home campaigns) in the 1960s, coupled with factors such as the increasing professionalization of the youth services sector, led to a shift from reformatories concerned with the 'normalisation' of inmates to a range of diverse provision, including foster care and smaller residential care units, and the expansion of socio-educational care (Hansbauer, 2008). The range of potential placement options internationally is varied and flexible, ranging from independent and semi-independent living arrangements, through fostering to residential, therapeutic and educational settings and secure accommodation or detention for children who pose a risk to themselves or others. Foster care now accounts for around three-quarters of placements in the US and UK (Children's Bureau, 2015; DfE/NS, 2016a) and is the most common placement option in Sweden, where large institutions have also been replaced by smaller group homes for adolescents and, often, provision for children under 13 to be placed with their parents (Hessle, 2013).

The last 30 years or so have also seen a rise in the use of kinship care (placement with close or extended family members or, occasionally, friends) across the developed world (Farmer and Moyers, 2008; Andersen and Fallesen, 2015). There are many recognized advantages of kinship care, which Lutman et al. (2009: 38) describe as often providing an 'enveloping supportive network', even where the placement itself is ultimately unsuccessful. These include less likelihood of stigma, greater contact with birth families, the commitment of kin, greater security of identity and ethnic and/ or cultural continuity (Sung Hong et al., 2011). But there are also widespread concerns, including safety; carers' age, health, low educational attainment and poverty; their use of or access to supportive services; and inappropriate contact with or pressure from birth parents (Farmer and Moyers, 2008; del Valle et al., 2011; Nandy and Selwyn, 2012; Coleman and Wu, 2016). Caregivers in Denmark, as in other nations, are poorly remunerated and given limited training and oversight (Andersen and Fallesen, 2015).

Social pedagogy in alterative care practice

Social pedagogy is both a professional and, in some places, an academic discipline, combining insights from social work and education (Kornbeck and Jensen, 2009). Originating in Germany, it is concerned with reflexive professional practice in the use of education (in its broadest sense) as a solution to social problems, through relationship-based practice with the whole child ('head, heart, hands'). Social pedagogy is well-established in much of Europe (Kornbeck and Jensen, 2009), including Slovenia, where it is a recognised profession (Kobolt and Dekleva, 2008), Sweden, Poland and Denmark. There is no universal understanding of social pedagogy as a theoretical or professional model (Eriksson and Markström, 2009; Hämäläinen, 2015; Janer and Úcar, 2017) and consequently its practice is characterised by considerable national diversity (Kornbeck and Jensen, 2009): Petrie and Cameron (2009) use the term 'social pedagogies' to reflect this. Modern social pedagogy in Germany supports both academic and biographical learning (the latter being defined as the way in which young people develop strategies to cope with their social environment) (Zeller and Köngeter, 2012). It is not a recognised profession in France, (although influential in Belgium, Switzerland and Québec, Canada), but there are some parallels with the French professions of 'éducateurs specialisés' and 'animateurs socio-culturels' (Bon, 2009). In Sweden, it has suffered from being of low status and poorly paid (Eriksson and Markström, 2009). Social pedagogy has only recently attracted interest in the UK, where its influence has generally been limited to early years and residential child care (Kornbeck and Jensen, 2009).

Despite the variety of social pedagogies, there are a number of common core principles, which may very briefly be summarised as a holistic approach to well-being, learning through supporting a child's innate potential, genuine and trusting adult-child relationships and empowerment of children to develop the skills for autonomy and citizenship (Kemp, 2011). Janer and Úcar (2017) report universal agreement that the functions of social pedagogy include social integration and the resolution of social problems, the promotion of social equality and social justice, and improving individual well-being and community cohesion. Coussée et al. (2010) describe social pedagogy as a perspective rather than a profession or method and warn that central to social pedagogic practice is critical reflection on the social context and its concern with individuals' relationship with, and integration into, society. This perspective arguably places social pedagogy in particular tension with recent Anglophone political discourses of individualisation and personal responsibility, yet care leavers' integration into and positions in society are a key concern of social policy in this area, as is considered in the following section.

Questioning assumptions about care and rehabilitation

The poor life outcomes of care leavers were briefly summarised in Chapter 1 and are discussed in greater detail in Chapter 5. On the face of it, statistics on a range of measures from mental health to employment, homelessness and incarceration, raise questions about the very concept of alternative care and reinforce its status as a measure of last resort. The reasons for the apparent universal failure of alternative care systems are highly complex and include deficiencies in support for young people ageing out of care, a primary focus of this book. But recent English research (Farmer and Lutman, 2010; Wade et al., 2010; Biehal et al., 2015) suggests that reunification is unsuccessful for most maltreated children, with 65 per cent of the 138 neglected children in Farmer and Lutman's study who had returned home no longer at home at the five-year follow-up and only a third of the 68 maltreated children in Wade et al.'s study having remained continuously at home after four years. In both studies, there were negative implications for well-being and stability associated with a further breakdown of the placement at home and for many children, exposure to further abuse and neglect in the home environment. Farmer and Lutman (2010) concluded that children aged over six when they returned home were less likely than younger children to achieve permanence in alternative care in the event that the return home failed. Similar arguments are being made in the Nordic context, where Pösö et al. (2014) question whether using out-of-home care only after extensive efforts to support the family have failed is in children's best interests. Put bluntly, privileging the right to family life may come at a long-term cost to children's welfare.

These observations reflect a broader problem in assessing the success of alternative care regimes. Ethical considerations preclude systematic randomised control trials on vulnerable child populations and, assuming assessment has successfully filtered children referred to child welfare services, those in care have experienced significantly more detriment than children in receipt of care services remaining at home. Moreover, a similar pattern exists in relation to different forms of alternative care: for example, although children in foster care in Denmark achieve significantly better educational qualifications than their peers in residential care (Andersen and Fallesen, 2015), this may say more about the population in each type of placement than the care itself. International comparisons are particularly problematic in this area because of the different forms of care and the range of welfare systems, together with a lack of systematic or recent data in many contexts (see e.g. Trede, 2008 in relation to the residential care sector in Europe).

The reality is that children in care are unlikely to achieve parity of outcomes with their peers without sustained support, not only during but also beyond childhood to compensate for the harmful effects of their pre-care experiences. State support for care leavers – a term generally used for young people aged over 16 who are in or have left state care – has developed since the beginning of the 21st century in recognition of the fact that these young people enter adulthood at a significant disadvantage to their peers. In the remainder of this chapter I briefly summarise the developmental tasks of adolescence and the contribution of Coleman's focal model of adolescence in explaining the particular challenges faced by children ageing out of care, before considering the contemporary context in which young people gradually attain independence in adulthood and recent developments in support for care leavers in developed nations. Finally, theoretical conceptualisations as to the basis for the state's responsibilities towards children leaving care are discussed in order to elucidate the rights which might be claimed against the state by young people ageing out of care.

Transitions to adulthood

The developmental tasks of adolescence

Despite the rapidly changing social context, the core developmental tasks of adolescence remain constant, and include physical (including sexual) and cognitive maturation, development of self-concept, achieving independence from parents and the foregrounding of peer relationships, including the development of intimate relationships (Call and Mortimer, 2001; Coleman, 2011). These developmental tasks are briefly outlined here because of the implications for young people who are required to understand their place in the social world and construct a theory of the self when not living with their birth parents and often while harbouring a strong sense of parental rejection and/ or of failure to meet parental expectations. Detailed discussion is beyond the scope of this book, but in basic terms, during adolescence children develop formal operational thought (the ability to understand abstract concepts and to apply logical reasoning to problem-solving) and make advancements in attention, memory, information-processing speed, information organisation and meta-cognition (the ability to reflect upon, plan and control cognitive processes) (Coleman, 2011). It is important to note that development of these skills is dependent upon external factors including the learning environment and perhaps the encouragement of significant adults (Coleman, 2011).

Adolescence is also a time during which social engagement expands beyond home and school (Call and Mortimer, 2001), in response to significant advances in young people's social cognition, with development of moral and political judgements and of 'adolescent egocentrism'. Adolescent egocentrism is a term used to describe young people's tendency to behave as though they are concerned with the response of an 'imaginary audience', which is assumed by the young person to have the same preoccupations – for example, their appearance – as the adolescent him- or herself. Associated with this is construction of the adolescent's 'personal fable', which elevates the individual's personal feelings to a special status and serves to bolster his or her self-concept during a time of rapid change (Coleman, 2011). Another key social developmental task of adolescence relates to impression formation, which enables young people to interpret the feelings and actions of others, distinguish their own impressions from those of others, and associate different behaviour with different situations, facilitating the making of new social relationships and appropriate conduct in group situations. In relation to moral reasoning, it appears that sensitive parental intervention, avoiding direct challenge but encouraging dialogue, may enhance development (Coleman, 2011).

As adolescents develop cognitively and physically, gain greater autonomy and encounter a wider range of social environments, so their self-concept develops. During this period, it is important for psychological maturation that young people make sense of the social world and their place within it, as their perception of themselves and their own agency will later significantly impact their response to life experiences (Coleman, 2011). According to Harter (2012), it is not until late adolescence or even early adulthood that young people are able to construct a theory of the self which meets the criteria identified by scholars in the field. Early adolescence (ages 11 to 13) sees a proliferation of multiple selves, which may cause distress through middle adolescence (ages 14 to 16), arising from an inability to resolve unstable or contradictory representations of self, particularly for girls (Harter, 2012). In late adolescence (17 to 19) young people develop a sense of possible future selves, associated with an increased sense of agency (Harter, 2012). In the modern world, Arnett (2000) concludes that identity exploration is primarily undertaken in 'emerging adulthood' (18–25) rather than adolescence.

Together with adolescent egotism, development of self-concept explains the preoccupation with self and introspection associated with adolescence. Self-esteem is an aspect of self-concept, regarded by Coleman (2011) as a good indicator of coping and adaptation. Parental influence is the most important factor in childhood, and although peers gradually become more influential from late childhood, the importance of parental support to self-esteem does not decline in adolescence: rather, parents and peers are influential in different domains, with parental support important in matters relating to school and family (Harter, 2012). It remains unclear whether success in school promotes self-esteem or self-esteem enhances academic performance, but the influence is domain-specific (Coleman, 2011): academic success alone will not provide self-esteem in other areas of young people's lives.

The focal model of adolescence

Although adolescence is still widely portrayed in the media as a period of turbulence, the 'storm and stress' theory of adolescence posited in the early 20th century was largely discredited by research showing that most young people negotiate adolescence fairly smoothly and maintain generally good relationships with their parents (Susman and Rogol, 2004; Coleman, 2011). More recent models include the lifecourse perspective, which seeks to understand human development through the main transitions and significant events or 'turning points' and is closely associated with developmental contextualism (a theory associated with Bronfenbrenner, among others) and the focal model put forward by Coleman (1974).

The focal model is based on empirical research demonstrating that young people cope with the developmental relationship demands of adolescence by 'pacing' themselves and tackling one issue at a time. Goossens and Marcoen (1999) have linked the model more explicitly to the process of individuation; that is, the way in which reliance on parents in early adolescence gradually gives way to separation from them in late adolescence. Other researchers such as Kloep (1999) have considered its applicability to a wider range of issues confronting adolescents. The model is used here because it posits that adolescents most likely to experience difficulty are those confronted with multiple challenges simultaneously (Coleman, 2011), which would include the vast majority of those ageing out of care.

Simmons et al.'s research in the US (1987) has endorsed Coleman's work in relation to early adolescents experiencing multiple life changes concurrently with the move to junior high school, demonstrating that multiple stressors are associated with a decline in grade point average for boys and girls and a reduction in self-esteem in girls. They use the expression 'arenas of comfort' to describe the importance of adolescents being able to draw on stability and comfort in at least one area of their lives or one set of relationships. This perspective enables focus on the sources of social support and protection of their self-concept available to adolescents, rather than on the stressors they experience (Call and Mortimer, 2001). Call and Mortimer (2001) suggest that relationships with parents are more significant in this regard than those with peers or in the workplace, but arenas of comfort outside the family can help to cushion negative effects of stress in the parental relationship. Girls report closer relationships with their peers than do boys (Call and Mortimer, 2001). These findings show little variance by socioeconomic status, although a higher socioeconomic background and a two-parent family is associated with a sense of comfort in more arenas of adolescents' lives, which in turn correlates to better mental health (Call and Mortimer, 2001).

The notion of arenas of comfort promotes attention to the way in which adolescents actively choose challenging or supportive social contexts and enables analysis of this process with regard to the macrosocial structures in which young people develop (Call and Mortimer, 2001). This concept of adolescent agency is central to the focal model: that is, young people actively construct their own adolescence, and their ability to cope with the transitional tasks of adolescence is attributable in no small part to the way in which adolescents shape their own adaptation (Coleman, 2011). The assertion that adolescents actively choose to resolve one issue before moving on to another is questioned by Goossens and Marcoen (1999) and Kloep (1999). Coleman recognises that young people do not have equal opportunities to control the way in which they manage their own development but concludes that those who are unavoidably confronted by many challenges concurrently are more likely to experience difficulty.

The focal model is relatively underdeveloped in the literature, and there have been no empirical studies testing it with 'non-normative' groups of adolescents (Hollingsworth and Jackson, 2016). However, it offers a powerful explanation for the particular difficulties faced by care leavers in their transition to adulthood, a process Stein has described as 'accelerated and compressed' (Stein, 2006a: 274), to capture the way in which English care leavers generally become independent at an earlier age than their peers, after a shorter transition period and with little or no opportunity to return 'home' should they encounter difficulties. A similar situation has been observed elsewhere, for example by Zeller and Köngeter (2012) in relation to Germany. Hollingsworth and Jackson's retrospective analysis of qualitative data from two previous studies (2016) supports the proposition that the concurrent negotiation of multiple transitions contributes to poorer outcomes for care leavers.

Education and social care systems both impose transitions upon care leavers, who may be concurrently grappling with significant personal challenges, including emotional trauma and educational deficits. Consequently, care leavers are likely to have limited control over the way in which they manage the developmental tasks of adolescence. They are likely to need more time than their peers to make a successful transition to independent adulthood, yet tend to be catapulted into independence at an earlier age. The focal model of adolescence explains the need for the creation of more normative transitions for young people leaving care (Stein, 2006a). Such transitions, for young people in general, have changed in recent decades to incorporate a more protracted journey to independence.

'Emerging adulthood': normative transition to adulthood in the 21st century

Adolescence has traditionally been regarded as a stage of transition from childhood to adulthood, but this view has been complicated in recent years by acknowledgement that not only does puberty start earlier than previously, but that greater engagement in further and higher education has delayed the age at which young people are able to attain independence from their parents (Furlong, 2009). These shifts have extended all three of the key changes of status traditionally associated with adolescence, namely the transition from school to work, gaining independence from the family and moving permanently out of the parental home (Coleman, 2011). Challenging economic circumstances, including relatively high levels of youth unemployment (Eurostat, 2016; OECD, 2017) and high housing prices, have exacerbated this trend. Consequently, there has been an increase in the proportion of young adults living with a parent or parents in the last 20 years, with the average age young people move out of the parental home now 26 in the European Union (European Commission, 2016).

For many young people, the transition to independence has become more complex and protracted, with traditional linear trajectories giving way to periods of 'backtracking' (Furlong, 2009: 1–2) and uncertainty (Heinz, 2009). Arnett (2000) coined the term 'emerging adulthood' to describe the period of instability typically experienced between ages 18 and 25. This new life stage is only available to young people in cultures which offer prolonged opportunities for exploration of potential roles and identities before committing to career and relationship choices. Young people identify a sense of responsibility for self, independent decision-making and financial independence as significant markers of achieving adult status (Arnett, 2000). While emerging adulthood is arguably a positive development in many respects, the instability which is characteristic of these years has been exacerbated by the recent economic downturn. Heinz (2009) draws attention to the tension between the expectations of a culture of individualism, which requires young people to give early attention to active decision-making to construct a meaningful biography in the context of insecure labour markets, and the extended transition to attaining independence described above. Care systems have been slow to acknowledge and respond to the ongoing needs of care leavers beyond the age of 16 and to adjust their support to reflect the implications of the status of emerging adulthood.

Support for care leavers

There is considerable variation in the ongoing support available for care leavers in young adulthood both within and between nations (see Stein, 2012, in relation to England), reflecting the fact that this is a relatively new area of social services provision in most. A review of Concluding Observations of the United Nations Committee on the Rights of the Child (UNCoRC) published in 2016 reveals that France, Ireland, Slovakia and the UK (UNCoRC 2016a-d) were all criticized for inadequate support and services for care leavers, while New Zealand (UNCoRC, 2016e) was censured for a lack of adequate data on children's health, education and well-being both in and after leaving care.

In England and Wales, acknowledgement of the inadequate support accorded to care leavers led to a specific legislative provision to extend the duties of local authorities. The Children (Leaving Care) Act 2000 created a complex scheme of staged support according to young people's age and care history. Thereafter, through the Children and Young Persons Act 2008, the Children and Families Act 2014 and the Children and Social Work Act 2017, policy has gradually attempted to provide a transition to adulthood more akin to that generally experienced by children brought up in their birth families. At the time of the CLET study, the local authority's duties (set out in s23 of the Children Act 1989 as amended by the Children and Young Persons Act 2008) persisted until the young person reached the age of 21, but young people continuing in education and training were entitled to financial assistance and other support from their former corporate parent to 25 (Children Act 1989 s23CA). Similar legislation has been passed in the US, where the Fostering Connections to Success and Increasing Adoptions Act of 2008 (P.L. 110–351) enables states to access federal funding to support young people ageing out of care to the age of 21, subject to their involvement in education, employment or vocational training. In Hungary, the Child Protection Act 2010 lowered the age to which 'aftercare' services are available to young people who do not continue in education. Young people may now leave care at 18, or can remain in 'aftercare' until they are 24 if they continue in education (25 if in full-time post-secondary education) but only until they are 21 if they are employed or seeking work (Rácz and Korintus, 2013). While most opt for aftercare, Rácz and Korintus concluded from their relatively small study that for most young people, there is no alternative, particularly for those that continue in education, although many had to contribute to funding their education.

Policies of this nature are intended to incentivise young people to continue in education – in some cases, Rácz and Korintus (2013) suggest, even when that course does not align well with their aptitudes and interests. However, they are liable to discriminate against some of the most vulnerable young people. Research has highlighted the value of higher education in facilitating a gradual transition to independent living (Stein, 2008), and young people leaving formal education early are likely to be less well-equipped for independence. In England, in response to such concerns, the Children and Social Work Act 2017 has extended the local authority's responsibilities to provide a personal advisor, needs assessment and 'pathway' plan to all care leavers under 25 if they inform the local authority that they wish to receive support and advice, and requires the local authority to offer advice and support to care leavers aged 21–24 at least annually (Children Act 1989 s23 CZB/s23CA-s23E).

Recent changes in England have also attempted to tackle the early age at which care leavers move to live independently, following US initiatives. Research on the operation of the US Fostering Connections to Success and Increasing Adoptions Act 2008 (Public Law 110–351) suggested that the benefits of allowing care leavers to remain in placements later more than justify the cost (Peter et al., 2009). Following a pilot study (Munro et al., 2012), section 98 of the Children and Families Act 2014 introduced a duty on English local authorities to consider arrangements for young people to remain in foster care placements until age 21 ('Staying Put') and to provide support (including financial support to foster carers) for such arrangements. To date however, the scheme has not been extended to children in residential care.

While provisions providing greater support to care leavers in young adulthood are welcome, they should not be viewed in isolation but must be considered in a social and economic context in which young people's transition to adulthood has become longer and more complex, as discussed above. Raising the age of compulsory engagement in education and training in developed nations provides an example of the state imposing extended dependency on its younger citizens. Such policies not only illustrate the blurred and shifting boundary between childhood and adulthood but also evidence the fact that this boundary may be differently constructed in different domains of young people's lives and that the factors influencing such decisions are often politically and socially determined, rather than being grounded in understanding of children's development and competence (Minow, 1986). The distinction between children's rights *qua* children and children's human rights becomes most significant at the cusp of adulthood and is of greatest import for the most vulnerable young people. The final section of this chapter therefore adopts a children's rights perspective in examining the state's responsibilities to children for whom it has taken over the parental role.

A children's rights approach to leaving care

The sources of the state's responsibilities to children in its care

Hollingsworth has identified four sources of justification for the state's responsibilities towards children leaving care through analysis of English documents and Parliamentary debates leading to the Children (Leaving Care) Act 2000 (Hollingsworth, 2013a). Of these, two – *generational* responsibility (the collective responsibility of adults for the nation's vulnerable children) and *equity-based* responsibility (drawing on the demands of social justice in relation to disadvantaged groups) apply fairly widely. The remaining two categories derive from the particular circumstances of certain groups of children. In relation to children in state care, the notion of *assumed* responsibility recognises that state usurpation of the parenting role carries with it an obligation to undertake that duty in the manner of a responsible parent. *Reparatory* responsibility acknowledges that the state has a duty to make amends to young people who have been let down by society in their treatment before and/or after entering the care system.

During childhood, the state actively limits the extent to which children may exercise autonomy and creates enforced dependency by children on their parents – for example, by requiring them to engage in full-time education and restricting their employment opportunities. Using a capabilities approach, Dixon and Nussbaum (2012: 576) argue that this dependency creates duties on the state to protect children from the risk posed by the consequences of decisions made for them, by 'insuring them against the risk that their parents (or legal guardian) will turn out to be unable, or unwilling, to take reasonable steps to protect their capabilities' – as is by definition the case for children taken into state care.

Reparatory responsibility validates the imposition on the state of ongoing parental obligations to young adult care leavers. The harm suffered by this group of children before entering care may result in an overwhelming burden in adolescence, often exacerbated by late entry into care. While the focal model suggests that young people typically tackle the developmental tasks of adolescence in an orderly and sequential manner, care leavers are hampered by far greater challenges which they are expected to overcome while concurrently negotiating transitions determined by society in education and social care. They have also been subject to early expectations of independence in societies in which their peers have typically enjoyed greatly extended family support during emerging adulthood. The significance of the leaving care provisions introduced in recent years lies in the acknowledgement that *de facto* autonomy at the age of majority may not be achievable for children in state care and the consequential creation of a duty on the state to compensate for that deficit in emerging adulthood. But in the context in which these duties have developed, they still leave children of the state with significantly less support than their peers.

A rights perspective articulates the justification of the state's reparatory duties more clearly. Underlying theories of moral rights is the notion that all persons are entitled both to equality of dignity and concern and to autonomy (Freeman, 1992). Eekelaar (1986) identifies children as having three broad hierarchical categories of interests: a 'basic' interest (in fundamental physical and emotional care and stimulation), a 'developmental' interest and an 'autonomy' interest. The notion of a 'developmental' interest posits that, subject to the social and economic circumstances of the society to which he or she belongs, everyone should have an equal opportunity to develop his or her capacities during childhood, such that he or she does not suffer disproportionate disadvantage upon reaching adulthood. Since fulfilment of this interest lies within areas such as health and education, for such an interest to be recognised as a legal right, it must be translated into duties through legislation and public policy. Writing in 1986, Eekelaar concluded that, save for the duty to ensure their children's education, parents in intact families are under no duty to fulfil their children's developmental interests, which for most children are also poorly or patchily protected as a right against the state in English law.

One example cited by Eekelaar (1986) of specific duties imposed on local authorities to meet children's developmental interests is that of provision for special educational needs. The duties owed to care leavers might be conceptualised as a right in a similar fashion: both groups of children require greater support than the majority of their peers if they are to fulfil their potential. Considering existing provision for care leavers from this perspective highlights a number of weaknesses, including the difficulty in enforcing poorly-articulated rights and, in some contexts, a discrepancy between the level of support offered to those young people continuing in education (and close to securing their capabilities) compared with those who are unable or unwilling to do so. Such analysis highlights the state's failure to offer equality of opportunity to some of the most vulnerable young people.

Eekelaar's concept of an 'autonomy' interest comprises a child's freedom of choice in relation to his or her lifestyle and social relationships. This interest must cede precedence to the child's 'basic' and 'developmental' interests in any circumstances in which they conflict, but should be fulfilled where possible without risk to the other two interests (Eekelaar, 1986). The 'autonomy' interest can be justified by reference to acknowledgement of children as people in their own right, notwithstanding their status of legal minority, but also by the fact that young people are subject to a presumption of full capacity to autonomous life as soon as they reach legal adulthood. Hollingsworth argues that this presumption should give rise to a duty on the state to ensure that the child is equipped for fully autonomous adulthood upon attaining legal majority at the age of 18 and has developed this argument in relation to children leaving youth custody through the concept of 'foundational rights' (Hollingsworth, 2013b).

The concept of foundational rights and its application to care leavers

Hollingsworth's concept of foundational rights makes an important contribution to the 'theory gap' in relation to children's rights, a term used to refer to the uncertainty which continues to surround the theoretical basis for children's rights *qua* children (Ferguson, 2013). The concept explains how children's rights are distinct from those of adults, through analysis of the difference between children's autonomy (as the basis in Hollingsworth's analysis for children's responsibility under the criminal law) and 'full' *de facto* autonomy exercised by adults. There has been some criticism of utilization of a rights framework in relation to child care work on the basis that, in a neoliberal political environment, rights tend to be posited on the assumption of the autonomous liberal citizen and to exist 'within a consumerist framework of legal relationships' (Smith, 2009: 11), overlooking the significance of personal relationships and social context in achieving the conditions required to achieve 'full' autonomy. One of the strengths of Hollingsworth's foundational rights framework is that it builds on recent work around relational interpretations of Sen's capabilities approach (Nussbaum, 2003; 2011), as well as Fineman's categorisation of 'social assets' (Fineman, 2008), providing a richer understanding of these conditions. 'Full autonomy' is distinguished from a narrower liberal definition of autonomy (comprising no more than adequate capacity to exercise agency coupled with freedom from external constraints on doing so (Hollingsworth, 2013b)) by the incorporation of recognition of the significance of relationships and social context in the identification and exercise of choice.

This wider relational conceptualisation of autonomy is particularly important with regard to children because of the primacy of parental and other personal relationships and of supportive social networks in achieving the developmental tasks of adolescence and in promoting resilient adaptation. Hollingsworth utilises accounts of autonomy as a relational concept in order to incorporate consideration of the way in which young people's relationships and social experiences shape their developing identities, and of the interaction between young people and their social worlds, which impact the choices available to young people and the way they exercise those choices. She does so by drawing upon the related concepts of 'capabilities', particularly as developed by Nussbaum, and of the 'assets' required for the development of full autonomy (a term used by Fineman, 2008, and Kirby, 2006) in relation to the concept of vulnerability.

Nussbaum's development of Sen's capability approach (Sen, 1979) stresses the importance of focusing on what people are able to do and to be – their 'opportunities and liberties' (Nussbaum, 2000: 71). Nussbaum argues that the concept of capabilities is instrumental in articulating what it means to assure to an individual a fundamental right, in that where a right is secured, a person is placed 'in a position of capability to function in that area' (Nussbaum, 2003: 37). Nussbaum (2000, 2003: 41) has identified 10 'central human capabilities', of which four are of particular relevance to this argument. The fourth capability, 'Senses, Imagination and Thought', includes

> [b]eing able to use the senses, to imagine, think and reason – and to do these things in a 'truly human' way, a way informed and cultivated by an adequate education, including, but by no means limited to, literacy and basic mathematical and scientific training.

The fifth, entitled 'Emotions', she defines as

> [b]eing able to have attachments to things and people outside ourselves; to love those who love and care for us.... Not having one's emotional development blighted by fear and anxiety.

The sixth, 'Practical Reason', requires '[b]eing able to form a conception of the good and to engage in critical reflection about the planning of one's life.'

The seventh capability is 'Affiliation', which Nussbaum describes as

A. Being able to live with and toward others, to recognize and show concern for other human beings, to engage in various forms of social interaction; to be able to imagine the situation of another.

B. Having the social bases of self-respect and nonhumiliation; being able to be treated as a dignified being whose worth is equal to that of others.

Nussbaum has developed three categories of capabilities: 'basic' or innate capabilities, which are present at birth; 'internal capabilities', which are acquired, primarily in childhood, and comprise 'trained or developed traits and abilities' (Nussbaum, 2011: 21); and 'combined' capabilities, which represent the interaction of internal capabilities with opportunities offered by the external environment in a way which enables the exercise of autonomy. Hollingsworth points to the particular importance of exposure to socialising environments in childhood, especially family life and school, for the development of a child's internal capabilities. Whilst parents are primarily responsible and influential in the development of the child's internal capacities, the social, political, economic and legal environment created by the state will impact on the external conditions which are relevant to the combined capabilities. For children for whom the role of parents has been assumed by the state, the state is the primary sphere of influence for both these sets of capabilities.

The assets identified by Fineman as being required for the development of 'full' autonomy are not dissimilar from the capabilities developed by Sen and Nussbaum and are those resources that society and state institutions must provide to mitigate vulnerability by enhancing individuals' 'resilience'. They comprise physical assets (such as material goods and wealth), human assets (given or developed capacities enabling an individual to acquire human capital, including health, education and employment) and social assets (supportive networks such as family relationships and community groups). Fineman (2008) uses the concept of 'assets' to argue in the US context for greater state responsibility for the way in which asset-conferring institutions such as education systems ensure equality in response to vulnerability. Her focus is on the way institutions may operate to reproduce power or disadvantage, rather than how multiple individual identities create or compound inequality. This provides an attractive approach through which to interrogate the reproduction of inequality in the lives of children in state care, both because of the heterogeneity of this group and because it draws attention to the attributes of state institutions which are directly responsible for these children's upbringing, such as the local authority 'corporate parent'.

Consideration of the significance of childhood in the development of the 'assets' required to achieve 'full' autonomy leads Hollingsworth (2013b) to identify a category of rights which support the conditions which will enable a child to acquire those assets, which she terms 'foundational' rights. She argues that the implication of the legal construct of childhood as a probationary period is that the state has a duty to ensure that children are equipped to exercise full autonomy on reaching legal majority, when the state removes the protection imposed during their childhood. The concept acknowledges the role of law not merely in regulating children's rights in recognition of their developmental capacity but also in promoting – or hampering – their development (Buss, 2009). Hollingsworth has developed the theory in the narrow context of the youth justice system, but its principles are equally applicable to care leavers because for this group of children, the state has not only taken on *assumed* responsibility (as in the case of young people leaving custody), but also holds *reparatory* responsibility.

Among the examples that Hollingsworth gives of the kind of rights that might qualify as foundational rights are two of particular relevance to the subject of this book, namely 'educational provision sufficient to develop the child's capacity for rational decision-making, as well as her future participation in political and community life' and 'protection of nurturing, positive, relationships that go beyond the prioritisation of certain *forms* of relationship to include also their *quality*' (2013b: 1062). These foundational rights map neatly onto Fineman's categories of human assets and social assets. They also reflect the interaction between a child's internal capabilities and the opportunities offered by the child's environment, in keeping with the concept of combined capabilities.

There are two particularly important implications of the concept of foundational rights for examination of the support offered to care leavers. First, it follows from the assertion that the state has a duty to ensure that young people reaching adulthood are equipped to exercise 'full' autonomy that, in relation to children for whom the state owes reparatory responsibility, the duty must extend beyond the age of legal majority, until such time as the young person secures the necessary conditions for the exercise of full autonomy. Second, the more vulnerable the child, or the further from securing his or her foundational rights, the greater the support he or she is entitled to from the state. Accordingly, the duties owed by the state to care leavers are not amenable to articulation by a 'one-size-fits-all' formula. Instead, they should be assessed on an individual basis, according to the particular needs of each young person and with regard to their individual exposure to risk and protective factors and the assets or capabilities required to assure to them their fundamental rights. Further, bearing in mind Coleman's focal model, regard should be given to the importance of enabling young people to confront challenges and transitions in their own timeframe.

Conclusion

Understanding the way in which care leavers' lives develop in young adulthood is complicated by the interplay of many factors (Allen, 2003), including the diversity of young people's backgrounds and experiences before entering and while in state care, as well as the social, economic and political environment in which they find themselves. While this group of young people are first and foremost negotiating a particular stage of human development common to all their contemporaries, the focal model of adolescence helps to explain why children parented by the state may require much greater support in the transition to adulthood than the majority of their peers. Modern care systems are beginning to adapt in response to emerging understanding of the experiences and needs of this unique cohort, but the support received by most still lags far behind that routinely offered to young adults growing up in their own families. Hollingsworth's concept of foundational rights not only provides justification for reversing this state of affairs but is particularly valuable for its attention to relational as well as educational aspects of children's rights. The following chapter examines the characteristics and experiences of the care population using insights from attachment theory before describing the personal experiences of the young CLET study participants in order to illustrate the interdependence between children's experiences of care and their educational engagement and outcomes.

3 The characteristics and experiences of children in state care

Diversity in vulnerability

Despite their different routes into care, the differing ethnicity and age profiles of children in care in different jurisdictions and the diversity of children's pre-care experiences within the care population of any state, as a cohort, children in state care share many similarities. Although data is patchy and definitions and measurements vary, the pre-care life experiences of children in state care are broadly comparable across nations. In their study of five European countries with different models of welfare provision (Denmark, England, Hungary, Spain and Sweden), researchers from the Young People in Public Care: Pathways to Education in Europe (YiPPEE) project found that study children from all nations, excepting unaccompanied or accompanied asylum-seeking children or immigrants, were likely to come from families with low socioeconomic status and have experienced a chaotic family life with separated parents, exposure to drug or alcohol abuse, crime, or parental mental ill health (Cameron et al., 2012). This chapter explores the research evidence on how maltreatment affects children and the implications of children's pre-care experiences for attachment to contextualise the pre-care experiences of the young CLET participants. The literature on placement stability and participants' accounts of their placement histories are considered, followed by discussion of the impact of children's pre-care and placement experiences on their education and school life.

The impact of maltreatment on child development and welfare

The effects of children's pre-care experiences on their development and well-being are potentially devastating. Child maltreatment is associated with significant mental and physical health problems, including greater likelihood of medical diagnoses and chronic illness (Hager and Runtz, 2012); atypical functioning in neurobiological processing, physiological responsiveness, emotion recognition and regulation, social information processing, school performance, and romantic relationships (Cicchetti, 2013); obesity and eating disorders; poor behaviour, including aggression; criminal conduct; and substance misuse (Gilbert et al., 2009b). Maltreatment affects a young child's self-awareness and ability to attend to his or her own wishes and feelings as a consequence of sustaining a state of hypervigilance to the actions of others. In older children, it results in negative self-perceptions which, in the case of chronic and severe maltreatment, may amount to a view of the self as despicable. Experience of maltreatment may also affect the integration of the multiple selves constructed during middle adolescence (ages 14 to 16), potentially resulting in dissociative identity disorder (previously known as multiple personality disorder) (Harter, 2012).

Repeated exposure to maltreatment over time and experience of multiple types of abuse exacerbate the psychological consequences, which are likely to persist into adulthood (Gilbert et al., 2009b). In addition to the implications for attachment considered below, children who have suffered prolonged periods of maltreatment may exhibit changes in brain function, associated with the effect of repeated stress responses, including symptoms of Attention Deficit Hyperactivity Disorder (ADHD), aggression and some types of memory problems (Glaser, 2000). Maltreated children, particularly those who are physically abused, are much more vulnerable than their peers to depression and suicidal ideation (Dunn et al., 2013). More severe abuse correlates with greater severity of depression and less improvement in depression over time (Valdez et al., 2015).

Physical abuse is associated with poor educational attainment as well as physical injury (Gilbert et al., 2009b). Childhood sexual abuse is associated with a wide range of adverse outcomes in adulthood, including mental health problems, symptoms of post-traumatic stress disorder (PTSD), sexually risky behaviours, physical illness and unemployment (Fergusson et al., 2013). Certain symptoms, including attempting to avoid reminders of the trauma, feeling socially detached and emotional numbness, have a particularly harmful effect on young people's social functioning (McLean et al., 2013), including the likely deleterious impact of insecure or disorganised/disoriented attachment patterns on future relationships (Harter, 2012). Neglect has received less attention than other forms of maltreatment but appears to be potentially as damaging (Gilbert et al., 2009b). Inadequate stimulation at sensitive periods of brain development may result in permanent damage to cognitive function, while insufficiently sensitive interactions with very young children may affect the development of the infant's self-regulation of affect, which may later manifest as aggression or hypervigilance (Glaser, 2000). Emotional abuse is associated with lower self-compassion in adolescence, increasing the risks of alcohol abuse, psychological distress, suicide attempts (Tanaka et al., 2011) and increased susceptibility to illness and lower life satisfaction in adulthood (Gavin, 2011).

Children in care are at greater risk of mental health problems, suicide and self-harm than their peers (Ford et al., 2007; Dubois-Comtois et al., 2015; Greger et al., 2015). A review of evidence from England and France (Stein and Dumaret, 2011) found that children in care in both countries suffered three to four times the incidence of mental health problems than their peers. Figures were worse for children in residential care than for fostered children. Stein and Dumaret's (2011) review suggested that mental health problems are likely to be exacerbated during the transition from care to independent living, consistent with findings that two in five English care leavers experienced deterioration in their mental health in the 12–15 months after leaving care (Dixon et al., 2006). UN Guidelines stress the importance of counselling and support during this transition period (UNGA, 2010).

Severity of maltreatment is associated with increased problems in externalising behavioural and adaptive skills (Jackson et al., 2014). Late entrants into care are less likely to achieve improvements in tests for inhibited attachment, social development and on the Strengths and Difficulties Questionnaire (Biehal et al., 2010), and they are more likely to exhibit problematic behaviour and perform less well at school than their peers who entered care at an earlier age (Sinclair et al., 2007; Dubois-Comtois et al., 2015). Dubois-Comtois et al. attribute the prevalence of behavioural problems among older foster children to the effect of prior maltreatment in the context of challenging developmental transition points, resonant with Coleman's focal theory (Coleman, 1974). Children's emotional, behavioural and mental health needs in care pose challenges for the provision of stable alternative care. Poor academic attainment of children in care and behaviour difficulties, including impulsivity and inattention, are correlated (Bernedo et al., 2014).

Using insights from attachment theory to understand the experiences and needs of children in care

Bowlby's theory of attachment has had wide-reaching influence on childcare practice because it shifted attention from physical care to the importance of emotional bonds (White, 2008). Bowlby's theory is based on the premise, drawn from observation studies of early interactions between mothers (and later, other caregivers) and their babies, that infants 'are preprogrammed to develop in a socially co-operative way': but 'whether they do so or not turns in high degree on how they are treated' (Bowlby, 1989: 9). The notion of a 'secure base' posits that the role of a parent in promoting a child's social development and emotional stability requires a child to feel encouraged to develop autonomy in the confidence that there is a reassuring welcome awaiting them from their attachment figure in times of stress (Bowlby, 1989). Accordingly, the sensitivity and responsiveness of the primary caregiver is regarded as causally related to attachment behaviour (NCCMH, 2015).

Attachment behaviour may be activated by young children's instinctive sense of fear, for example when left alone or when experiencing an unfamiliar environment. This behaviour varies according to the child's condition (including ill health and tiredness); the whereabouts and behaviour of the attachment figure; and the wider environment around the child and may range from checking on the attachment figure's whereabouts to clinging and crying. Separation from the attachment figure induces separation anxiety, a term used in a wider sense to cover the perceived unavailability of the attachment figure. A child's attachment figures are usually hierarchical: different attachment patterns may develop with different adults, with children exhibiting a strong preference for a particular individual. Attachment behaviour develops between the ages of six and 18 months and is clearly exhibited until at least the second and often the third year when the child begins to recognise the primary caregiver as an independent person, enabling a more complex relationship to develop (Prior and Glaser, 2006). But these dynamics are significant throughout the life course, such that attachment behaviour, simply explained, leads individuals to maintain closeness to another whom they regard as better able to cope (Bowlby, 1989). In adolescence, parental attachment figures begin to give way to peers, and in adulthood, to partners or close friends. In old age, there may be a reversal of roles such that the elderly parent's attachment figure is an adult child (Prior and Glaser, 2006).

An infant's attachment strategies may be organised or disorganised. Three types of organised attachment behaviour (now usually referred to as secure, insecure- (or anxious-) avoidant and insecure-resistant/ambivalent) were identified through the Strange Situation test, in which the responses of infants aged nine to 18 months to unfamiliar surroundings, the departure of their carer, the introduction of a stranger and reunion with their carer are observed (Ainsworth et al., 1978). A fourth category of attachment behaviour, insecure disorganised (or disoriented), was later added by Main and Solomon (1990) to account for infants whose behaviour is contradictory or appears disoriented or incoherent. Disorganised attachment is considered the strongest indicator of poor long-term outcomes (NCCMH, 2015).

Key parenting behaviours to promote secure attachment include consistent, prompt, sensitive and benign responsiveness to the child's signals and comfort when the child's attachment behaviour activation levels are high. Intrusive or rejecting parenting is associated with insecure-avoidant attachment; unpredictable and/or poorly-involved parenting with insecure-resistant attachment; and a 'frightening or frightened caregiver' with disorganised attachment (Prior and Glaser, 2006: 55). The nature of the interactions experienced by a child are also significant in their contribution to the 'working model(s)' that the child constructs of the attachment figure(s) and him or herself in relationship with them. Bowlby (1969) considered that attachment patterns in the early years owe more to the particular relationship with the attachment figure and are open to adjustment should the caregiver's conduct change, but as the child develops and the working model is built, the attachment pattern stabilises. Good communication with and from parents enables children with secure attachments to update their working models more readily than can insecurely attached children (Bowlby, 1989). These working models influence the child's self-concept and relationships outside those with the attachment figure(s). Where the attachment is disorganised, the child constructs multiple inconsistent internal working models in response to perceptions of grave risks to the self, resulting from current or previous experiences of abuse or loss (Joubert et al., 2012).

The association between maltreatment and attachment

There has been relatively little research specifically investigating the association between child maltreatment and attachment patterns (Stronach et al., 2011) and even less on the attachment of children in care (Bovenschen et al., 2016). Around two-thirds of attachments in the general infant population across cultures are secure (Prior and Glaser, 2006), but Cicchetti et al. (2006: 636) found secure attachment to be 'virtually nonexistent' in their sample of 137 maltreated infants. A higher incidence of insecure attachment and particularly disorganised attachment has been found in maltreated children compared to their peers in a significant body of research (Glaser, 2000; Stronach et al., 2011; Harter, 2012), including in relation to foster children and their carers (van den Dries et al., 2009; Bovenschen et al., 2016). Disorganised attachment appears to be a better indicator of child maltreatment than the 'toxic trio' of caregiver characteristics (substance misuse, domestic violence and mental ill health) (Wilkins, 2012).

Crittenden's work (1988; 1992) suggests that abused children develop an internal working model based on hierarchies of control and power, which protects them in the short-term through compliant behaviour with the abusive adult and dominance towards siblings, but militates against their ability to make trusting relationships in the longer term. Neglected children, in contrast, come to see themselves as helpless; their resulting passivity reinforces their internal working model of the unresponsiveness of others. Where children exhibit severe and persistent abnormal social function associated with attachment behaviours, they may meet the criteria for diagnosis of an attachment disorder (American Psychiatric Association, 2012; World Health Organisation, 2016). In the first systematic study of Reactive Attachment Disorder (RAD) behaviours in 153 non-institutionalised adolescents who had experienced early familial maltreatment, Kay and Green (2013) found that over half the high-risk sample scored significantly higher than the control group on a range of measures of RAD behaviours.

The implications of attachment behaviours for the care of maltreated children

Secure early attachment is significantly associated with adaptation in early childhood (Easterbrooks and Goldberg, 1990) and good functioning in later years (Prior and Glaser, 2006), including communication, cognitive engagement and mastery motivation in school (Moss and St-Laurent, 2001); sociability with adults and peers and compliance with parents (Greenberg et al., 1993); and situational adaptation of impulse and emotion (Easterbrooks and Goldberg, 1990). It also plays a role in buffering the body's physiological response to stress as evidenced through cortisol elevation (Prior and Glaser, 2006). Securely attached children are likely to display less aggression than those with insecure-anxious attachment, although children with insecure-resistant attachment may perhaps be less aggressive than securely attached children (Savage, 2014).

Insecure attachment in early childhood correlates with emotional and behavioural difficulties later, with clear associations between insecure-avoidant attachment in the early years and aggressive or anti-social behaviour and negative affect in later years; and between insecure-resistant attachment in young children and withdrawn, anxious and passive behaviour when older. Children who have suffered maltreatment and exhibited disorganised attachment before moving to live with alternative carers are likely to exhibit a range of behavioural difficulties, including aggressive, coercive or controlling behaviour towards carers (Prior and Glaser, 2006). Disorganised patterns are predictive of symptoms of depression in middle childhood (Bureau et al., 2009). They are also associated with aggression and delinquency in adolescence and with anger, aggression or violence towards partners in close adult relationships (Obsuth et al., 2014; Rholes et al., 2016). RAD behaviour is associated with severe social impairments, including disruption to relationships, self-care and adaptive functioning (Kay and Green, 2013).

Childhood attachment is a mediator between child maltreatment and a range of adult outcomes (Muller et al., 2012). Achievement of secure attachment with mothers and peers is associated with less problematic emotional and behavioural functioning among young adult survivors of child maltreatment (Lowell et al., 2014), while adult attachment style is regarded as a potential mechanism in explaining the propensity for risky behaviours. Emotional and sexual abuse are associated with both anxious and avoidant attachment styles in adulthood (Oshri et al., 2015). Attachment anxiety predicts both psychological aggression and victimisation in adult romantic relationships (Rholes et al., 2016) and is positively related to alcohol use, while avoidant attachment is positively associated with drug use and antisocial behaviour (Oshri et al., 2015). The effects of emotional maltreatment on internalising, externalising and trauma-related symptomatology in young adults is partially mediated by attachment style in close relationships (Muller et al., 2012).

Cognitive capacity may also be affected by attachment issues. Joubert et al.'s US study (2012) of 60 adolescent mental health patients with a history of maltreatment found unresolved/disorganised attachment to be significantly associated with dissociative trauma symptoms and with poor working memory, but not to affect verbal or thinking capability, in keeping with other work suggesting that disorganised attachment leads to a tendency for attention difficulties under stress. Working memory was found to be a mediator in the relationship between unresolved attachment and trauma symptomatology.

The 'attachment state of mind' of foster carers also appears to be signifi-cant in predicting behaviour difficulties in foster children (Prior and Glaser, 2006). This term is used to describe adult attachment patterns through cat-egorisation according to the Adult Attachment Interview (AAI), namely as autonomous-secure, dismissing-insecure, preoccupied-insecure, unre-solved/disorganised or cannot classify. Dubois-Comtois et al. (2015) found that quality of interactions was a significant predictor of children's behav-ioural difficulties, although the direction of this relationship could not be confirmed. Lower levels of commitment towards the child were found in preoccupied and unresolved foster mothers than secure-autonomous moth-ers. A far higher proportion of foster mothers were categorised as having an unresolved attachment state of mind, in keeping with literature that suggests that their own childhood adversity may prompt people to become foster carers. This finding is concerning because an unresolved attachment state of mind is associated with cognitive difficulties, including in the self-regulation of cognitive activity (Joubert et al., 2012). Unresolved or cannot classify styles of adult attachment predict significant parenting difficulties and disorganised patterns of attachment in the child (Murphy et al., 2014).

A comprehensive review of the international evidence base on attachment in children at risk of or in care, or adopted, concluded that the quality of the evidence for interventions is low (NCCMH, 2015), but research suggests that effective interventions for attachment are often similar to traditional parenting interventions in their focus on parenting skills and the quality of child-parent interactions: parental sensitivity and consistency is key to secure attachment (Chaffin et al., 2006; Wright et al., 2015). While it was neither appropriate nor possible to explore the attachment styles or interactions with carers of the young people participating in the CLET study, the summary of relevant literature here is intended to provide a contextual framework to the following accounts of the young people's personal histories.

The personal histories of the young participants to the empirical study

Loss, bereavement and rejection

The 21 young people in the study came into state care between the ages of four and 15. 12 did not enter care until after they reached secondary school age. The majority of the group was in care due to maltreatment or fam-ily dysfunction. Three were or had been UASC: Riley had been remanded into care; Devora was a British orphan; and Ollie was in care because he had significant physical and mental disabilities. The circumstances of many were complex. For example, Habib had entered the country with his family as an asylum-seeker, but his parents suffered mental health problems, and he had also been diagnosed with ADHD (Attention Deficit Hyperactivity Disorder).

Only a few had experienced stable and consistent care from a young age, including Michael, Ollie and Devora. Michael had Asperger's Syndrome and had been with his foster carers since he was four: they would have adopted him but for the consequential loss of support from the local authority. Ollie had been cared for in a residential home for disabled children for most of his life, and he would continue to be dependent all his life. Devora, an only child, had lost her mother as an infant and her father when she was 13. Her life with her father had been greatly circumscribed:

> he was so over-protective of me that I couldn't even go to sleep-overs... or parties... Yeah, my social life, I have one now...I had to do all the housework and look after him, and that's not a childhood...I think I started doing the housework...like five or six years old.

The three asylum-seeking young people had had to come to terms with loss of their wider community and way of life, as well as their family and friends. Farouk remembered travelling with a woman who brought him and two siblings to the UK:

> I didn't know her, she came with us here and then she left us...at a chicken shop, and she said she would be back, and she never came back. Went outside, and we was lost, we didn't know what to do...we found someone who speak our language, and then she took us to her home, and we stayed with her for a little bit, then she called the social worker.

Bashir explained:

> My brothers and sisters...I don't know where they are, because...my granddad's sent me and my cousin to this country just for protection, but...father I don't know where he is, this five years I don't know where my mother is...and when I came to this country I treated my foster carers like my new parents, because I knew I'd lost them, there wouldn't be any way back to find them.

When asked what, if anything, she would change in her life, Sofia said simply: 'I just need my mum and my family, that's all.'

Loss, bereavement and rejection were key themes of the personal circumstances of the cohort as a whole. Riley had lost his best friend in a house fire, while Ollie's father died during the course of the study, as did one of Habib's carers, triggering difficulties in his relationship with the remaining carer. Tasmin's father had died when she was seven or eight, following which her mother's drug use had worsened. Tasmin had taken on much of the care of her brother, who was then a baby or toddler, and she described finding it 'really hard to let go' of that parenting role when they were taken into care, albeit together. Priya entered care at the age of 13, when she was pregnant, but had not been able to keep the baby, who it appeared had been removed

from her care. For Devora, her orphanhood seemed to be far more significant than her care status:

> *are there any other looked-after children in the school?...*
> I don't have a clue...I know there's quite a few of us that have lost par-
> ents, a parent...I can go to them if I feel low, and if I just need someone
> to talk to that knows what it feels like.

Not long after her father had died, Devora's best friend had started to ignore
her, and she felt quite alone: 'I have friends. Yeah...Not as close as I want it
to be though. I don't know if that's because of my circumstances'.

The principal sense of loss concerned young people's relationships with
their birth families. A sense of rejection continued to impact most of the
young people many years after their entry into care. At least two of the
young people gave accounts suggesting that they blamed themselves for
their removal from their families. Habib seemed reluctant to attribute cul-
pability to his birth parents for their neglect:

> ...it was kind of my fault that I was in care, because a social worker
> came knocking on the door and...there was me and my younger sib-
> lings, and I opened the door, and she goes are your family home?....and
> then after that they got on my case...that's something in my memory
> that sticks out...That was when I was like six.

Adam had decided not to pursue the relationship with his birth family:

> I don't think they are really bothered, because there's been several times
> they could have arranged to meet me at a secure place...and they've just
> left it for about five years, six years...
> *So you haven't seen them for a while?*
> No, I don't need to too, I don't think I want to...I don't want to see
> any of them no more.

Kayla had attempted to meet up with her father, whom she had not seen
since she was six, but he failed to turn up for two arranged meetings:

> I'm not really bothered with him anymore...First time it was...some-
> thing to do with a job, second time he was running late...he was sup-
> posed to come at two thirty, we waited until seven thirty and he still
> didn't come...And he said he wanted to see me...

Habib had not seen his family for about eight years and was more forceful
in expressing his feelings:

> I feel pissed off...My dad, I don't know him, I don't care. My older
> brothers, I don't care, I don't like them, I don't associate myself with

them. There's been enough times, yeah, they were meant to come to contact, and it's not a thing where they couldn't come...They were just too lazy. So why should I give a fuck with them if they don't give a fuck with me? Sorry.

Jacinda described her mother as 'a bit dodgy', saying she 'stopped talking to me, which is quite bad...I couldn't really trust her, because she lies a lot, so I don't really know the truth from her any more'. Gilroy was insistent that he attended the school he was at because his father had wanted him to attend a Catholic school, but he had not in fact seen his father for four years: 'whenever we plan a meeting to go and see my dad he's never in, he's always gone away or he's out'. When asked 'if you could do anything at all with your life, what would it be?' he replied 'see my family more maybe'. Elliott said he saw a lot of his family, but: 'obviously I would like to go back to live with my mum, my granddad or something, with my family, but...I'm in care, it's alright really'. His mother was invited to relevant meetings – 'she comes sometimes, but sometimes she doesn't come'. Ollie's sisters still lived at home with his mother; he too would have liked to go home, but thought 'she won't let me live with her because she thinks I will hit her, but I won't hit her'.

The importance of sibling relationships to children in care is recognized in research and policy (McBeath et al., 2014). Separation from and poor contact with siblings is a source of distress for many young people (Herrick and Piccus, 2005; Wojciak et al., 2013). Maintaining relationships with their siblings was particularly complicated for some of the young people in the CLET study, many of whom came from large and/or separated families. Qadira and Kayla were both one of seven children; Adam had three sisters, one in foster care with him, one living independently and one in foster care in his home borough. Imogen had an older sister at university and a younger one with learning difficulties, who had been adopted: she had contact with the younger one, but her mother did not. Callum had a brother and sister living with his father a considerable distance away, and he had lived with another sister until she was moved:

> I used to see her every day and now I don't see her at all....she got moved to a care home because of her behaviour, drugs all this stuff, then I think she was causing trouble in that care home...she got moved to...some place really far out...Haven't seen her for months, long, long time...don't think now we are not even allowed to call her, only certain times, she's not allowed to have a phone.

Jacinda and Habib had particularly changeable relationships with siblings. Jacinda had three brothers. The eldest had been adopted, and she only met him towards the end of the study after he had found and contacted her through Facebook. The middle brother had been in foster care with her before moving to live with his father when she was seven, but he was later removed to a different placement. The youngest was also in a different placement; he was moved to another and then returned to Jacinda's mother during the study. Habib had four siblings. Four were originally placed together but split when Habib's older brother wanted to move, and Habib left with him. At that stage he was 'really attached' to his elder brother but 'wasn't really attached' to the younger siblings, who since moved to live with his elder sister. Later, when his older brother wanted to move again, Habib had stayed in his placement, now alone. By the final interview, his relationship with his older brother had become more problematic: his brother was dropping in and out of college and Habib was trying to persuade him to attend ('I tell him. I tell him to go'). With hindsight it appeared that Habib thought his brother's behaviour might have had much to do with his own ('I might of got influenced'). By then, he thought the most important people in his life were his younger brother and sister, then in their mid-teens ('I love them to death'). He arranged contact himself now that he was over 18, but he was only able to see them about every half-term.

When I first met Kayla, she no longer saw her mother, and she only saw her sister twice a year because she was 'not reliable'. Only Kayla's youngest brother was in the same foster care family as her, as an older brother had moved out at 16. She would not see him until her younger brother felt able to because he had been aggressive. Two siblings had never entered care, one of whom was in the US, and another brother had gone to a residential children's home. During the study, one of her brothers came out of prison, but social services would not allow the youngest brother contact without their oversight. The older brother would not agree to their involvement. Kayla had met him once, but 'it was kind of weird because I didn't know what to say...like starting off again'. These kind of complexities compounded issues of placement stability.

Placement instability

Placement instability is considered a key risk factor for attachment difficulties (NCCMH, 2015). It appears to be associated with disruption in the development of the prefrontal cortex of the brain and correlates robustly with poorer outcomes for care leavers in young adulthood (Vinnerljung and Sallnäs, 2008; Fisher et al., 2013). Biehal et al.'s study (2010) comparing outcomes for adopted children with those in long-term foster care highlighted that emotional and behavioural difficulties are unlikely to improve until children are in stable, long-term placements. Moreover, placement breakdown (Rock et al., 2015) appears to predict a raised risk of placement instability thereafter. Van Santen (2015: 195) uses the term 'placement careers' to describe the pattern of disruption that may develop as a result of children's experiences of multiple placement moves. Care leavers with placement career histories are at statistically significant greater risk of substance misuse even than their peers ageing out of care, after controlling for a range of background adversity variables (Stott, 2012). They are also more likely to experience hospital care for mental health problems, have no more than basic educational qualifications, be dependent on social welfare and be sentenced to probation or imprisonment for criminal offences in young adulthood (Vinnerljung and Sallnäs, 2008).

In England, around two-thirds of children experience only one placement in any year, and 10 per cent experience three or more (DfE/NS, 2016a). In the US, most children are in care for a relatively short period, but those in care for more than two years are likely to experience significant placement disruption (Pecora et al., 2006). In Stott's study of 114 young adult care leavers, the average number of placements was eight, amounting to a move on average every six months: nearly one-fifth of the sample had experienced 12 or more placements. Although the evidence base suffers significant limitations (Holtan et al., 2013) Olsson et al.'s conclusion (2012: 13) that 'unplanned placement breakdowns...appear inherent in the out-of-home care phenomenon itself' is supported by studies from the Netherlands (van Rooij et al., 2015), Germany (van Santen, 2015), Spain (Bernedo et al., 2015), Norway (Christiansen et al., 2010) and Denmark (Olsson et al., 2012).

Child risk factors for premature placement termination include (externalising) behavioural problems; diagnosed medical conditions, especially of emotional disturbance; perceived mismatch with foster carers; ethnicity; age; separation from siblings; poor relationships with biological children of foster parents of a similar age; and prior unsuccessful placements (Oosterman et al., 2007; Courtney and Prophet, 2011; Khoo et al., 2012; Fisher et al., 2013). The relationship between difficult behaviour or mental health problems and breakdown appears complex, but is likely to be bi-directional (Stanley et al., 2005). Bernedo et al. (2014) found the warmth of foster care to be an important positive factor in placement stability in their Spanish study. Foster carers who place a high degree of importance on supporting children's academic attainment and development of life skills may promote a sense of stability and confidence, thereby enhancing placement stability (Rock et al., 2015). Teenagers should be actively involved in placement planning as they are unlikely to tolerate a poorly matched placement, and more intensive support for their placements should be provided in the first year, when disruption is most likely (Olsson et al., 2012). These findings may in part explain why experience of multiple social workers is also associated with increased placement instability (Rock et al., 2015).

Some research has found a lack of understanding of the demands of fostering, lack of tolerance towards the children in their care and unrealistic expectations among some foster carers (Hyde and Kammerer, 2009; Christiansen et al., 2010). Adolescent participants to Hyde and Kammerer's qualitative study of placement moves (2009) stressed foster carers' lack of expertise in responding to the grief and anger children exhibited. Studies universally suggest foster carers would benefit from greater advance knowledge of a child's needs and support from social services (e.g. Khoo and Skoog, 2014), particularly for older children (Olsson et al., 2012; Bernedo et al., 2015). They also highlight foster carers' concerns as to the inadequacy of training and support to help them cope with difficult young people, especially when there is a crisis (Harkin and Houston, 2016); concern over the risk to their family or the foster child from violence is a key consideration in carers' termination decisions (Brown and Bednar, 2006).

Breakdown instigated by both children and foster carers is more likely as children grow older, but girls are more likely to instigate placement termination than boys (van Santen, 2015). The primary foster parent risk factors are parenting stress (Farmer, 2010; Khoo and Skoog, 2014; van Rooij et al., 2015) and professional concerns as to the standard of care (Beckett et al., 2014), as well as external events such as carers' separation. Foster carers are more likely to terminate placements of male children, children joining the family due to behavioural problems and children placed between six and 15 years old (van Santen, 2015). Racial discrepancies in placement stability remain largely unexplained, but the greater instability experienced by African American children in the US may in part be accounted for by a greater preponderance of risk factors such as emotional and behavioural problems; higher rates of disability and special educational needs; and low socioeconomic status (Foster et al., 2011). Asylum-seeking or refugee children appear slightly more likely to achieve stability than their peers (van Santen, 2015).

Although children placed with kinship carers have sometimes been found to experience better stability than those in non-relative placements (Courtney and Prophet, 2011; Font, 2015), other research casts doubt on these findings (Lutman et al., 2009; Andersen and Fallesen, 2015). Farmer's study (2010) suggests a greater commitment and willingness by kin carers to persist with the care of very troubled children, but unplanned termination was more likely among kinship foster placements than stranger care placements in van Rooij et al.'s study (2015) in the Netherlands. Contact with children's birth family appears to be an important factor for stability of placement, but the evidence is mixed (Rock et al., 2015). Overall, high quality contact appears to be associated with stability of placement, but other factors are more influential, and placement breakdown is more likely in cases where contact is problematic, poorly planned or unsupported, particularly for children with a history of maltreatment (Sen and Broadhurst, 2011). Adequate supervision of parental contact is particularly important in relation to kinship placements (Farmer, 2010).

In the care of strangers: young people's experiences of care

Placement (in)stability

Unfortunately, the CLET study participants' experiences of placement stability mirrored the literature. Table 3.1 shows the number of placements experienced by participants and the last known placement, highlighting changes anticipated in the near future.

Table 3.1 Young people's placement histories

Name	Entry into care	No. of known placements	Last known placement	
			Since (age)	Type
Adam	9/10	3	10/11	Foster care (awaiting council housing)
Bashir	12	2	12/13	Foster care (intending independent at end of school)
Callum	12	3	17/18	Independent (council housing)
Devora	13/14	1	13/14	Kinship care (awaiting council housing)
Elliott	11	1	15/16	Foster care
Farouk	11/12	4	17/18	Independent (with elder brother)
Gilroy	12	4	17/18	Custody
Habib	9/10	5	17/18	Supported accommodation (awaiting council housing)
Imogen	8/9	'loads'	17/18	Semi-independent (awaiting council housing)
Jacinda	6	At least 4	9	Foster care (until finishes uni.)
Kayla	5/6	2	9	Foster care (until end 1st year uni.)
Luis	6/7	2	13/14	Foster care (prob. stay post-18)
Michael	4	1	4	Foster care (will stay post-18)
Niall	12/13	About 5	17/18	Semi-independent (didn't attend housing panel)
Ollie	?	1 or 2?	?9	Residential care home (ends at 18)
Priya	13	About 6	16	Supported accommodation (ends at 18)
Qadira	12/13,	4	16	Supported accommodation (awaiting council housing)
Riley	15	3	16	Supported lodgings (awaiting council housing)
Sofia	16	2	18	Independent (council housing
Tasmin	8	4	13/14	Foster care
Unity	11	About 10	16	Supported accommodation (ends at 18)

Young people were eloquent about the reality of living as a stranger in other people's family unit. Some failed to settle in care at all and deliberately disrupted their placements. Unity said:

> Obviously they are strangers. They just dump you there, 'there you go, there's your new placement', you don't know no-one, you are in the middle of nowhere, and it's a bit daunting.

Kayla thought treatment of the foster children in one of her placements was 'really disturbing. We weren't allowed in the living room...because their sofas were white...we just didn't want to be there, so we all played up...We couldn't handle it...we were treated completely differently'. Priya declared 'I don't like living with strangers'. She deliberately sabotaged a foster placement: 'I told them that I wanted to move, and social service don't listen...so I gave trouble so I could move'. Qadira had liked one of her foster placements until a new girl came, with whom she 'didn't get on': 'we had a fight, and then I just took my stuff and moved'.

Others described a pattern of short-term carers, failure to get on with foster families and differential treatment from carers' birth children. Luis thought he had changed carers because the first carer was not providing an adequate standard of care. Imogen described 'loads' of carers from the age of eight to nine before remaining in a stable rather than happy placement from age nine to 17. Gilroy's placement had also seemed stable initially, but he chose to move to semi-independent accommodation, saying only 'I moved from there...Didn't like it...Got bored with it'. Riley had no notice of a move from one care home to another: 'they literally turned up and said right, you're moving, pack up your stuff'.

Jacinda experienced a number of short placements between the ages of six and eight, before she settled into a permanent placement. Although she was very happy in the first placement, it was short-term and she was required to move:

> I just didn't fit in, I didn't like it. I guess because I really liked the family that I first moved in...and then I got moved to another family and I just didn't want to be there, so I was a bit of an annoying child.

In one of the short-term placements, she said

> the parents' daughter...used to like hit me and my little brother, like kick us around...And she used to make us sit up and watch scary movies...I watched Scream when I was only six.

Tasmin also attributed her behavioural shortcomings to her experiences in foster care. She was cared for by four families from the age of eight to 16. The first was short-term; the second lasted four years but ended because the carers had 'family issues'; she was very unhappy in the third, and explained

'I was really badly behaved...I was with one that I didn't really like, so I was always angry'. Her pleas to be moved were ignored until the carer became pregnant. She had been with her current carer, with whom she had an excellent relationship, for two years when we first met.

Unity found it 'stressful' living with carers: 'they used to give me orders telling me I can't do this, I have to do this, I have to do that...Like what time I had to be in. They used to ring police, report me missing'. Unity was angry to have been moved out of her home area, to keep her away from influences thought to be harmful to her. She thought she had experienced about 10 placements, consistently running away (and therefore enduring four periods of secure accommodation) until she eventually settled in the last, back in her home area, in which she remained for 15 or 16 months. That provision stopped at 16, when she was placed in supported accommodation. Priya also moved to supported living arrangements at 16, following placements in four care homes, in which she claimed to have been assaulted, for a few months each. Riley had attended two residential homes and the contrast was dramatic. In the first, he said:

> I spent more time with the police and in hospital, they just weren't looking after us properly...They just done their own thing and left us to it, they weren't keeping an eye on us, they weren't helping us cook, they was just letting us be, run around like idiots should I say – which we were.

Riley's designated teacher Ms Coral endorsed his view of that home, which she described as 'diabolical'. The second was 'a lot better...staff just made you feel like it was your home, they looked after you, they done things with you, they talked with you. Helped me when I needed it' (Riley). At 16, the residential home was no longer available, and Riley moved again, this time to supported lodgings with a couple who were police officers, which worked well for him.

Relationships with carers

Only a few fortunate girls (Jacinda, Kayla and Tasmin) appeared to have the kind of relationship with their carers that could be regarded as being as close and supportive as one would expect from birth parents, but these relationships were invaluable. Tasmin said of her foster carer, 'I go to her about everything to be honest'. However, this placement was under pressure from her brother's behaviour for which Tasmin thought her carer was not getting adequate support, particularly since his counselling sessions had been stopped by the local authority: 'She finds it really hard...his behaviour's really bad. He's like a bull'.

Jacinda genuinely felt part of her carers' family: 'I've been with my family for so long I just don't feel I'm in care now'. When asked who she thought were the most important people in her life, she unhesitatingly replied 'family, my mum, I call her mum'. While she attributed this strong relationship to the length of time she had been with the family, it was also clear that they treated her as they did their own children, including taking her on holiday with them to Thailand soon after she came to live with them. She said she thought she was 'one of the lucky ones in care' because her family is 'so lovely'. Jacinda knew she had a family for life: 'they always say that I'm part of the family, they say if I do want to leave I can, but they'll still be there if I want to come back, that's what they all say'.

Similar promises had been given to Adam, Tasmin and Kayla. In his first interview, Adam said he wasn't 'really bothered' about his birth parents' rejection because 'basically they [his foster family] are my family now', adding 'my carer said because she's so nice I can stay with her until I want'. Tasmin said that when she had told her carer she might want to go to university, 'she was like "I'm always here for you", so that's good'. Kayla reported that although the leaving care team said she would have to leave care at 18,

> my carer said I can stay until they think I'm ready, *I* think I'm ready to move out...if I wanted to come back, I can always come back...I was happy when they said that.

Promise of an ongoing relationship was especially important to Kayla, whose early history had resulted in her finding it difficult to make personal relationships with her peers and particularly with boys. She felt that her foster father and brother had been extremely instrumental in enabling her to overcome those difficulties, adding 'I think it will get better as I grow older, and I'm still in contact with my carers. If I'm not I think...I'll retrack a bit and just go back how I was'. For Kayla, this placement, where, she said, 'we are loved', was the best thing about her experience of care: 'I think just being with them has made me settle down, and I know that my family is there for me'.

Jacinda, Kayla (sometimes) and Michael were the only participants to refer to their foster carers as their 'parents', but even very stable placements such as Michael's tended to have a fragile quality. Michael expressed significant anxiety over 'taking the strain' off his parents and a sense of a reciprocal rather than unconditional relationship with them:

> Like if there's any way that...I could help, I do it...They've had us since we were four and six, it's about time we started...helping them... because if they get upset about stuff we've done I just don't like seeing them upset....

Only two of the young people experienced kinship care, Devora, who named her cousin as the most important person in her life ('without her I'd probably be in the care system, God knows where, loads of foster carers or in a home') and Callum, who lived briefly with kinship carers. Callum was much happier there than in his previous placement, and felt he had made significant progress:

> ever since I moved in with my auntie I've done well at school…I was still bunking some lessons, but…I coped much better in school…I'm more mature…They've helped me a lot…they've changed me…acting like I'm a seventeen-year-old, you know, not acting like an idiot…

However, this placement had broken down by the time we met for the last time, and he was living independently.

Imogen only confided in the final interview that she had not had a good relationship with her foster mother since she was 10 or 11, although she had 'got along' with the rest of the family, which in part explained why she had stayed. Matters came to a head when the carer locked her out (seemingly not for the first time). Imogen ran to her mother's where she stayed until semi-independent accommodation was found for her. She said she loved living on her own because 'I don't have people saying [Imogen] can you do this, [Imogen] can you do that'. When asked whether there were any changes she would like to see in the care system, Imogen replied 'I think they should like really look into who they pick as carers'.

In Habib's case, realisation that he was treated differently from his carers' birth children dawned gradually as he grew up. In his first interview, Habib described himself as 'happy' in his placement, but by the final interview, the relationship had broken down. Habib felt that he was treated less favourably than the carers' much younger son, adding:

> I was with them for like five years or something…they've decided to let me go and they've never like even texted me back, so…I have their number…but I ain't gonna really do eff…for people who don't care about me so…don't really care to be honest.

Even where relationships were good, participating young people – like many adolescents – might not feel able to confide in their carers. Luis described a good relationship with his carers, who were the second family he had lived with, and with whom he had lived since about age 13, shortly before he was excluded from mainstream school. When asked if he felt that either of his carers could have supported him differently, he said 'I'm not sure actually, I didn't tell them lots of stuff'.

The interdependence of care and education

There were two key consequences of the kind of personal difficulties described above. The first related to the effect of placement disruption on educational continuity and the second to young people's ability to engage in education. This section provides an account of young people's educational histories in care, including educational disruption and difficulties before considering professionals' views on supporting young people's engagement in education and helping them achieve their potential.

Educational disruption

Many of the young participants had missed substantial periods of education and/or experienced several school changes. Habib had entered care when he was nine or 10 and described an unsettled home life:

> My dad...he never taught me, I didn't really know how to speak properly...I went to school, but I was like...in, out, in...I kept moving houses...I never stayed in one place, I never stayed in one school...Probably twelve...I can remember a lot of schools I went to.

Adam, too, moved around a lot when living with his mother:

> probably about seven different houses...I've been all around London, I know every part...Not getting taken to school...I probably...started school properly in Year 6 [age 10–11].

He described the effect on his education:

> I was 'what is all this?' I couldn't even say ABC...the teachers was teaching all the other people...I didn't have a clue. I was just sitting there...I couldn't do one plus one, I couldn't write my name.

Both Qadira and Unity described attending primary school regularly but encountering difficulties adjusting to secondary school. Unity, who entered care at 11, explained 'last time I was like permanent in school properly was primary school...and when it was secondary it went pear-shaped, my life went off the rails'. Qadira found secondary school 'boring' and was excluded for assaulting a teacher. By the time she entered care at 12 or 13 she was registered at a Pupil Referral Unit and appeared to have an entrenched aversion to school:

> Schools haven't really been my thing, like. Can't explain it, but...I just don't like sitting in the classroom and listening to people telling me what to do.

Sofia, Bashir and Farouk had entered the UK from Angola, Afghanistan and Somalia respectively. Sofia had learnt English at school and experienced regular school attendance in her home country, while Farouk had had a limited home education before coming to England. Bashir explained 'I didn't really go to school much there, and I think it's very different...the education is not very good there'. Both boys knew only 'a bit of English' (Bashir), on arrival, but coming to England provided opportunities not previously available to them, and as with many asylum-seeking young people (Jackson et al., 2005; Jackson and Cameron, 2012), Bashir, in particular, was determined to make the most of his education.

Once in care, the established association between placement disruption and educational difficulties (O'Sullivan et al., 2013) became apparent, with changes in school resulting from placement moves and behavioural difficulties. Although Habib was clear that his educational opportunities had been improved by entry into care, he had had a far from ideal experience, attending at least five schools from four foster placements.

Riley entered care through remand at the age of 15 and missed most of that academic year through a combination of factors, including late school placement on moves to each of two residential homes followed by an inability to adjust to school:

> I lasted three hours over two days in one school, and then I got moved to the [Pupil Referral Unit]....I just didn't cope, I had a fight, almost had a fight with a teacher...We got arguing and he threatened me, and that's it, I just kicked off...It was just the way I was.

For Unity, school moves arose directly from her inability to settle in placements:

> I left school quite young. I went to a number of different schools, but never really attended...Obviously when I run away from placement and then they'd move me and it was all big confusion...
> *How long did you manage to stay in a school?*
> ...only a few months at a time, but I never really attended...wasn't happy where I was, so was rebelling, didn't want to go to school...I went to two different secondary schools...and I went to a few like PR [Pupil Referral] units, went to three different...four different ones, done a bit of home schooling.

In general, local authorities endeavoured to avoid placement changes when children were studying for public examinations at 16, in accordance with statutory guidance (DCSF, 2010). However, the extent to which representation from the virtual school was included in placement decisions varied. Virtual heads considered that they were not always consulted appropriately. In Ironbridge, young people were often brought back into the local authority from therapeutic out-of-borough placements at 16, a process in which there was 'no consultation...whatsoever' (Mr Steel). Ms Mason recounted a young person being moved from a residential home into another area a few weeks before their examinations, and sitting none at all as a result, although they had been predicted to do 'really well': 'it wasn't the sort of crisis that couldn't have waited a little bit longer...we were not part of the decisions'. Such examples highlight the value of the virtual head holding a position of seniority within the local authority and wielding influence in both social care and education to ensure that decisions take into account all aspects of a young person's life.

Ms Mason had experienced children being moved into semi-independent accommodation at 15, a practice she described as 'madness'. Mr Brook acknowledged that resource implications played a part, explaining: 'sometimes...a placement will change from foster care to semi-independent because...the young person is just not making use of the foster placement, and...that foster carer could be...working with another young person'. But Ms Oak at Forest Hill College described a young woman whose behaviour had deteriorated to the extent that she was facing exclusion, seemingly triggered by a move from foster care into hostel or semi-independent accommodation: 'the type of young person she is, the other young people that will be in there, I don't think she will do well in that environment, but... we are one voice around a table of many'.

Educational engagement

While many of the young people had behavioural and/or school engagement difficulties prior to entering care, for some, including Niall and Callum, the distress associated with the events leading to their entry into care manifested in disruption at school on entering care. Five of the 12 boys had been ex-cluded from school or college (Gilroy, Habib, Luis, Niall and Riley). Some young people were more articulate than others in describing the challenges they faced in adjusting to school, but it is important to consider briefly young people's accounts of their difficulties in conforming in school and engaging in their education. Callum explained:

> before I went into care I was in Year 7, and the whole year I was great, I was brilliant, no bunking, nothing, I was amazing that whole year...I was down when I went into care...from Year 8 to Year 10 I was non-stop bunking, swearing at the teachers, doing bad stuff.

Although Callum had made considerable progress since entering care ('I did calm down a lot in Year 11'), his personal history continued to impact on his educational career. He had missed a lot of school since entering care and was facing criminal charges for an offence of violence when we first met, an incident for which he narrowly avoided exclusion through the good offices of his designated teacher.

Many of the young people referred to similar difficulties in behaving con-formably in school, and in particular keeping their temper. Gilroy consid-ered that it was helpful for staff to know his care status 'in case people say things about my family...I try and keep...calm, but if they keep going on and

I lose my temper they'll know why…and they'll understand'. It was not only young people's behaviour that was affected by their care histories, but also their ability to concentrate and learn at school. As Priya put it: 'I'm smart, basically it's that a lot of things were going wrong for me when I was doing my GCSEs and I couldn't concentrate'. Gilroy appeared to associate his dislike of school with the fact that he had entered education late:

> I've tried hard at it, since I've been in school, but I've never liked it…I joined primary school in Year 4, so I missed the whole…basics of school, so I'm learning; I'm trying to catch up.

Adam gave a powerful account of how difficult he found secondary school for a significant period after entry into care:

> we went to [the learning support unit] and the teacher would teach us how to spell, write, count, and all stuff like that…it would just confuse me…I did work hard, but I was just not learning, but all of a sudden your brain just clicks. It's weird how it happens…because in the beginning it just goes out of your head, what goes in comes out.

Eventually, however, it all came together, and to his great credit Adam achieved very good GCSE results, saying: 'My brain feels like it's there, and my head feels like it's on my shoulders now'.

Similarly, when discussing placement moves, Tasmin explained 'I wouldn't be able to concentrate, and like my mind would wander, and I'd be like worried all the time, so kind of like had an effect on my education…I'd always be in trouble'. This affected her relationship with some teaching staff:

> I used to dread coming to school on days I had teachers that I didn't get on with, because I was like "I can't be bothered" for that lesson…And like I find it really hard to control my anger, like I get angry, and then I'm angry for ages, and I just like won't talk to anyone.

Although Tasmin's own anger had resolved now she was settled in her placement, her brother's behaviour affected her ability to study to the extent that she considered moving in with her sister: 'I want to stay with him but he puts so much pressure when I'm trying to do work, I want to focus on my studies'.

For a few young people, such as Priya, who was out of education, training or employment throughout the period of the study, the outstanding issues in her personal life appeared to preclude her being able to engage at all: 'it's not like I don't want to go into education, my life just needs to be sorted out properly first before I can deal with something like that'. Priya's explanation resonates with Coleman's focal model of adolescence, as does Adam's. See also Ms Tan's account of a young person whose mother had rejected him for 12 or 13 years before taking him back home when she had addressed her own problems:

> ...[he] reverted back to being about four years old...he went from focusing on getting GCSEs to being absolutely focused on needing his mum. So he was about six foot four and...couldn't bear to be away from her...I've never seen such a dramatic turnaround...he needed to resolve those issues far more than getting an education.

Kayla similarly acknowledged that her school work had suffered when she first turned 18 and had focused attention on her family relationships:

> I was struggling in the beginning...because I was able to see my family, and it was like confusing me with my schoolwork, everything was just getting too much, and now that I've balanced it out I've managed to be on top of my work.

The difficulties recounted above were acknowledged by professional participants. A significant advantage of the virtual school system was evidenced in enhanced communication to schools about the background and needs of new entrants into care and creating better links between social care and education. Professionals highlighted the fact that children entering care aged 12 or over were likely to have a history of instability in their personal lives and their education, including considerable involvement in and understanding of the procedures leading to their entry into care. As a result 'they are a lot angrier' (Ms Lea) and 'there are all kinds of things that need to go in first before there's going to be any kind of fruitful learning or engagement' (Ms Mason). Some young people 'couldn't really engage in education, let alone exams, at all' (Mr Brook). Professionals also recognised that behaviour at school was often much less challenging than behaviour in the placement, and it was important for the school to be supportive of carers: 'the fact that they get them in the taxi and get them to go to school is a major battle, and that's the one to win...and sometimes I'll say to them "let school deal with the school issues"' (Ms Teal).

Ms Olive taught GCSEs over one year where possible, to try to ensure that where there was disruption during the two years leading up to them children still left with some qualifications. She was head-teacher of a school for children with social, emotional and behavioural difficulties (SEBD), with many children placed out of borough (The Grove). Two 15-year-olds had recently left the school after making unauthorised contact with family members through technology, in this case Facebook. In one case, the child was so distressed by the information they uncovered that there were violent incidents at home, resulting in two emergency foster placements and a return to his birth family, no school placement at all during his GCSE year and reported involvement in drugs.

Other designated teachers in non-mainstream schools reflected on the inherent tension between focusing on social and behavioural issues – without which educational qualifications would remain inaccessible to young people – and the importance of qualifications for success in adult life. Ms Tan explained:

> I want children to be able to read and write, to be able to realise that education is a way forward to make their lives completely different...But actually leaving with five A-Cs is neither here nor there, what it is for them is...to be in a position where they can access adult life, and make some real, positive, choices.

Ms Carmine, who ran a small independent PRU, was aware of the need to ensure a viable pathway post-16 if young people were to have a chance in life. Although she started out focusing on 'hands-on skills for life', she quickly concluded that she needed to aim for young people to get the qualifications to enable them to access college. She too, however, acknowledged that supporting young people to obtain qualifications was only a part of the work that she did and that it was about more than a passport to the next educational stage:

> ...sense of achievement, just improvement on their outlook on life really...it's not just about getting them to the end, the whole child really, you've got to think about, there's emotional development, social development.

Conclusion

The very individual nature of young people's experiences before and in care, coupled with the complexity of their lives, renders any single theory inadequate to explain their conduct and their choices. Additionally, young people's attachment status was not assessed in this study. As a consequence, I have chosen to present the young participants' accounts in this chapter in a way which allows them to speak for themselves, supported by some evidence endorsing the key themes from professionals' examples of similar stories. Yet the very real consequences of maltreatment and attachment difficulties are vividly apparent from these accounts, together with evidence of the way in which placement difficulties compound the challenges young people are already facing.

A number of issues come through clearly from these accounts. The first is the importance for children in care to have a sense of family belonging and of being valued and loved by carers. Related to this is the enduring value or importance of birth family relationships to young people, which perhaps helps to explain the challenges faced by the care system in replicating a sense of 'real family' for children in state care. Second, it is apparent that there are emotional as well as practical barriers to engagement in education for many young people and that Coleman's focal model of adolescence goes some way towards illuminating these challenges, but they are complicated by children's pre-care educational experiences. The importance of education in the lives of care leavers and the evidence base on improving educational outcomes for children in care are discussed in detail in Chapters 5 and 6. Finally, Bowlby's description of attachment across the life course as expression of the need to feel able to rely on someone better able to cope during times of adversity has significant implications for care leavers and was acknowledged by Kayla in her prediction that if she loses touch with her foster family she is likely to 'retrack a bit'. The support of a consistent, reliable and caring adult is a significant protective factor in resilient adaptation and requires particular attention as young people transition from care to independence. Resilience is the final theoretical lens employed in the book and is considered in the following chapter, which provides a more detailed consideration of the implications for children's personal lives and education of being parented by the state.

4 Children of the state

Corporate parenting in principle and practice

Introduction

It is apparent from the accounts in the previous chapter that providing children with a placement in which they can genuinely feel part of the family unit is challenging and may perhaps become more so as young people progress through adolescence. However, the status of being in state care and the practical consequences of the state holding parental responsibility or exercising parental functions held far wider implications for young people's relationships and experiences in school as well as in their personal and home lives. This chapter first explores the experience of 'being in care' and of 'corporate parenting' and the impact on young people's daily lives from the perspectives of both young people and professionals, including issues of stigma and trust; surveillance and bureaucracy; and impersonal and transient relationships with social workers. The cumulative effect of these experiences is analysed through the concept of self-reliance, widely regarded as an aspect of resilience. The notion of resilient adaptation and insights from the 'coping' literature are employed in order to consider the ways in which the resilience of children in care and care leavers might best be promoted. In the final section, the congruities between the theoretical lenses of attachment, resilience, the focal model and foundational rights are reviewed to draw together findings on the importance of relational aspects of the lives of young people ageing out of the care system.

Being in care

Status, stigma and stereotyping in school

Most, but not all, of the young study participants were reluctant for their care status to be widely known (see also Harker et al., 2004), which limited the extent to which they could be open with their peers. Adam, for example, said that none of his friends knew he was in care, although he had by then been in care about five years. He thought most of the teachers knew. Gilroy said:

> I only tell people who I know will keep secrets, and I can really, really trust...there are two kids I really trust in this school, that I told, but it's like other people I won't tell them nothing about my lifestyle.

The girls often described only telling their 'close friends' (Tasmin, Imogen) or 'best friends' (Kayla). Jacinda said 'I told my best friend, but the others don't need to know', while Priya told none of her friends at school. Participants were concerned that they would be treated differently by peers and/or staff, a common finding in the literature (e.g. Honey et al., 2011):

> I don't want to feel like I'm out of the ordinary…I want to be treated as an equal (Devora).
> I want to be like the same, I don't want to be different (Imogen).
> I don't want to be treated different compared to everyone else (Elliott).
> I don't think hardly anyone knows that I am, I don't kind of like to show it off to anyone, because I don't know, I'm sometimes scared they might treat me differently, but everyone thinks I'm just like them, so it's good (Kayla).
> Everyone has this negative stereotype of people that are like in care…I know quite a few people…are nothing like the stereotype, and one of them's working and got an apprenticeship…and doing really well…the stereotype's really annoying and it sticks to you through life as well… Yeah, I think most of them kind of like stick to like near care as well, doing care work I noticed, a lot of them go back to being social workers or foster carers or like counsellors…Yeah, I don't fit that stereotype, it's quite annoying, it gets on my nerves (Tasmin).

Michael used his foster carers' surname rather than his birth family name and went so far as to deny being in care if people asked, saying 'they don't know at all. If they do say that I say "no", I deny it…if they know I'm in care they might treat me differently, they might use it as an excuse to bully me'. Callum, in contrast, had been open about his care status and suffered the consequences:

> They know…Don't mind that…They used to take the Mick ages ago, when I first told them…Saying that my mum didn't want me, stuff like that…They said they were joking about it, they don't do it anymore, so…

Callum later explained that he had not been allowed to see his mother for some years and that she had self-harmed. Understandably, school taunts in such circumstances were more than he could handle: 'that was an excuse to bunk all my lessons and I used to get angry and get into loads of fights, you know, people'd say something about my parents'.

Those who did not mind others knowing their care status were effectively already singled out through their education or placements. These included Niall, one of only nine boys in his private alternative education provision; Qadira, who attended a number of pupil referral units (PRUs); Habib, (also in a PRU) who said simply 'some of them know…it's not an issue'; and Riley, who was in residential care and said: 'everyone knew I was in care; it doesn't bother me that people know'.

Most of the young people accepted that some or all of their teachers needed to know their care status, and that it brought them additional support, but would have preferred for them not to have been told. Priya said: 'every teacher knew my business, and that's why I don't like it, I like things to stay private'. When asked if she thought teachers needed to know, Jacinda said 'Not really. It's the past...I guess I don't really mind, but...it's weird knowing that all the teachers... know your business'. She had taken steps to ensure she was not singled out:

> At first when they had all the...meeting it used to be in school and I used to be pulled out of class, and everybody would be like 'what happened, what happened?' And I used to feel like the attention was on me, and I complained, and after that they decided to do it after school...I think they should do that with other children in care. Then they'll feel like they fit in, instead of having to be pulled out of classes and people asking questions and you don't want to answer them.

For the most part designated teachers in mainstream schools were sensitive to the importance of respecting young people's privacy but recognized that this could affect the way in which they were able to undertake their role. Mr Green described his experience at Fairfields:

> most of the time they really don't want to talk to me, understandably so...they are really, really resistant to talking about it...I spent a lot of time talking to [Elliott] in the week, we had a dance show on, and he'll talk about anything, and when I asked him if he'd do this [the interview] I was really amazed that he agreed...but he just doesn't want to talk about it with *me*...We had one go to university last year...who absolutely would not speak to me. I mean again she would talk to me about anything [else]...She wouldn't attend PEPs [Personal Education Plan meetings], didn't want anything, just came in and got on with her work, and I think she got three straight As in the end.

Ms Willow at Millbank College recounted her experience of a young woman on whose account she had been called to a meeting:

> They want to be like everybody else, and not be isolated for any reason...I went down to her, and I called her out...She was quite clear "I'm not going to discuss it with you"...And I've only ever seen her in passing again...and she looks at me and you can see that look of fear come over her face, and I just go "hi, how are you doing", and walk on. But there's that fear, because she's told no one, not even her tutor...and I think if you inadvertently destroy that confidence you do far more harm than good in a way.

Most schools had arrangements in place to try to avoid singling young people out in front of their peers, to ensure that they did not need to interact with multiple staff members and to make available to them members of staff with whom they were most likely to feel comfortable. Since the designated teacher role is held at a senior level, this generally meant taking advantage of pastoral systems within the school or of administrative staff with whom young people came into contact in any event: in Fairfields and Clifton, this was often the attendance officer, or 'just whoever they latch on to' (Mr Green, Fairfields). Ms White, Ms Teal and Ms Gold stressed that they tried to undertake their role as discreetly as possible:

> I think most of them prefer it if I stay out of their way, because they don't like to be identified as being different, so I'll only meet them if I absolutely have to...I mean usually the contact that they would have would be mostly with their head of year (Ms White).
> support needs to be discreet...And I know in some schools the designated teacher will meet very, very, regularly with students to see how their progress is. I suppose my view on it is that I will assess and establish and revisit things as and when I feel it's the right time (Ms Gold).

At Woodhall, Mr Brown said that 'they know that I'm the person who will keep a general overall eye on them, but their first contact will be their form tutor, their head of student learning'. Similarly, Ms Coral stated:

> it was kind of very low key really, it was sort of like a watchful eye... from a distance, rather than me meeting them regularly...their tutors would have taken responsibility for them, just like any other child...but they were all made fully aware who I was, and what my role was, and that my office door was always open.

Queen's had recently appointed two non-teaching pastoral leaders, who managed the PEPs, including ensuring that students completed their parts of the form, while at Garden House all students had achievement mentors, whom they called by their first names, and they would normally tell the mentors if there were any issues they wanted to raise.

Nonetheless, young people's sense that their personal lives were public property within schools appeared to be borne out to a significant degree. Schools varied as to the extent of information that was shared, but most regarded it as important that all staff were aware of which children were in care, so that teachers understood the children's circumstances and allowances could be made if necessary:

> at the beginning of the year we have an inset day, and I make all staff aware who the looked-after children are, and how to manage them, I suppose, in their behaviour, and if there are any issues with their education that they should contact me. And I do that regularly...because teachers do sometimes forget, and don't realise that there's other issues

surrounding a child's education...sometimes dealing with a looked-after child might be different to dealing with another student, you know, in terms of confrontation, and keeping in touch with a carer, and letting me know as well (Ms White).

One of the big roles I've always thought I have is to explain our children to the teachers, because lots of our teachers are very young, very inexperienced (Mr Brown).

Everyone knows, so on their registers they will know who the looked-after children are in their class (Ms Rose).

We publish the register of students who work with learning support, and we also publish the list of vulnerable students, so staff are aware of where the pressures are and which students we are monitoring and tracking in specific detail (Ms Gold).

Schools appeared to take a paternalistic attitude to information-sharing, which in most cases was not something young people had any control over or knowledge of:

I see myself as being the advocate for that child inside the school... you are like the extra parent...if that child is not doing well you will talk to the teachers. But the child themselves will not be aware of that (Mr Brown).
And do children get any say in the matter?
We don't ask them...when we mention it to staff, we do say...this is not something we want you to address with the student...But we feel it's quite important, because they need to know the family circumstances... not *why* they are in care, but *that* they are in care, and so when you speak to them it won't be mum or dad, it will be a guardian, and sometimes they are taxied in and out as well, so arranging after-school detentions and things is not as straightforward as it might be with ordinary children... And also containing that information...I don't think everybody needs to know why that child is in care, and what the issues are. That's confidential, and I think the more people that know those things the less confidential it is (Ms White).

I have an hour, every September, at the beginning of school...where I would introduce new students to school, and it's only three or four who are the most challenging,...so we have two looked-after this year...I did have a lot to explain what the circumstances were, what the issues are, how they can help them out...if there are very specific things that are happening in their lives we have a good system of communication with their pastoral leaders, and then we would let them know what's happening, and it would be passed on to teachers, as much as they need to know, that maybe in this particular period she might be slightly unusual, so just bear that in mind, there is something else going on (Ms Rose).

Mr Green summed up the impossibility of avoiding disclosures that would be unwelcome to young people:

> I think we are pretty honest with them. But...they just don't want the staff to know...we'll say to them "who do you need to tell? Who do I need to tell about this?" And they say "no-one". And I say "I need to tell Miss [X], I'll tell [the attendance officer] because she's easy to get hold of, and kind of knows these things, and I'll tell your tutor, and I'd like to tell your teachers". And they'll say "no"...if you try and involve them in it they just don't want anybody to know, which is fair enough.

Colleges appeared more likely to respect confidentiality, with Ms Willow observing that although she would ask young people if they would mind her sharing their status with their teaching team, she would generally respect their wishes if they asked her not to 'because I think at the end of it they need that respect, they need to know that we will respect their wishes'. Instead, she might flag up with staff, with the students' agreement, that she was working with a student, so that they were aware that they should contact her before taking action on an issue themselves.

In non-mainstream schools it appeared usual for all staff to know the child's status, but because of the nature of the institutions, this was less likely to cause them to stand out from others:

> there will be children who are given more one-to-one than looked-after children, more social interaction, because they need it because of their educational needs...we don't think 'looked-after child'...they just happen to be looked-after children...But what we do with them in school, and how we kind of support the families, isn't limited or expanded, the fact they are looked-after or not (Mr Grey, special school).

Surveillance, intrusion, and bureaucracy at home

The unwelcome sense of being subject to a greater degree of scrutiny than their peers at school was mirrored for many young people in their home lives. Unquestionably, there is a need for foster care to be monitored by social services and this was illustrated in the case of Niall's carer, who Ms Carmine felt was unable to offer adequate care and whose status was revoked by the local authority during the course of the study. She said:

> The carer that he's with is not an official foster carer...It's from when he went to a school called [x], he was friends with one of the students there, and it's a parent from there...it's kind of an unofficial basis, but they've left him there...basically, I'm just picking up the pieces.

However, the level of surveillance was a source of considerable frustration for some young people. Qadira stated she disliked her first social worker 'because she was just too much in your business, I don't like that'. Monitoring arrangements appeared to be especially problematic where foster carers were employed by a private agency which was then overseen by the local authority. Tasmin was particularly outspoken on the subject and wished that her foster carer could be given greater control over day-to-day decision-making, something that has since been introduced. Whether this will reduce the level of surveillance felt by young people like Tasmin, however, is uncertain:

> she has to write notes every day about us, and it's so annoying...Just like what we've done in the day, if we've been bad, or like if we're rude...I feel like I'm in the Big Brother house...it's like she's checking up on us every day...And she was like 'well I can't not write them', she has to follow procedures, and I know, fair enough, but I still think it's a bit rude that they make her do it. I feel like I'm being watched all the time. It's ridiculous.

When asked about the issues student care leavers were most likely to come to her about, Ms Willow at Millbank College cited difficulties in placements, often to do with perceived surveillance, including young people who were not allowed to use their mobile phones unless in the hearing of the foster carer, on loudspeaker, where there were constraints on contact with their birth family.

Devora and her carer, who was her cousin, decided to apply for a Special Guardianship Order (SGO) to discharge the care order and end the local authority's involvement. Devora said 'she's just fed up with all the paperwork that they give her that she has to do for me, and it takes up all her time doing all that work, it's just really stressful for her'. Devora was not many months short of 18 before the order was passed, partially because the process started before she transferred to the leaving care team, and was disrupted by that move, which itself was delayed until she was over 17.

Delay could cause considerable difficulties for young people at this time in their lives. Priya blamed missing out on a place at college on delay in her post being forwarded from her former foster carer to her new accommodation because she obtained her acceptance letter after the date on which she should have attended the induction day, while Jacinda nearly missed a holiday because of difficulties obtaining her passport. Imogen had been unable to see her birth family for 'quite a while' because she was waiting for social services to arrange it: Jacinda, in contrast, after her experiences with the passport, had taken matters into her own hands to ensure that she saw her mother on her birthday ('they just took so long, and in the end I just did my own ticket, sent them an email of my ticket telling them how much it was, and then went up myself'). Farouk and Devora both had to wait a considerable length of time for social services to apply for a National Insurance number to enable them to obtain work. Farouk felt left in limbo when his college registration was revoked because of his immigration status, and he could not even join a local football club without the local authority's agreement. There was very little he could do with his time and he was feeling quite low in that interview, explaining:

> I know they've gone low [his footballing skills], I've put on weight as well...I used to play football nearly every day, that used to keep me fit. Now I'm having to go on my own and like jog around the park and all that, and sometimes I go football for a different club...I asked my social worker if I can join, but she's taking a long time to get back to me...It's just extra-curriculum so I don't know why it's taking so long...you have to pay for registration, and like when you go training you have to pay two pound, and the match is two pound as well.

Callum was involved in a road traffic accident, following which he needed to take a taxi to school. When I met him for his second interview, he had only started back at school that week, although he had wanted to return two or three weeks earlier ('because I knew I was missing such a lot of work'), but his social worker had not made the necessary arrangements until then. Kayla's laptop had broken down in January of her last year of school and had still not been returned to her when we met at the end of March, so she had to write all her coursework out by hand. Jacinda had needed to prove her care status to obtain the bursary from her college but was at the time between social workers:

> they were saying that they needed a letter, and I was messaging the manager at social services, and they took so long, so I ended up just taking a load of old letters that proved I was, and then eventually they believed me.

Often, the source of frustration lay in the fact that it was difficult to obtain timely (or any) responses to requests, yet social workers appeared to undertake many tasks that seemed unnecessary to young people, visiting or completing administrative tasks for no specific purpose other than regular monitoring. Imogen said 'they always give you this form that you have to fill out, always, all the time, and nothing ever happens'. Riley tolerated rather than drew support from contact with his personal advisor, which she initiated 'normally when she wants to get something done', such as a review meeting or consent to disclose information. He said of his experience of social workers, 'all they do is come out, not very often, see how you are, and that's it, go away again...they don't do anything'.

Over time those young people that I interviewed on more than one occasion became more open about things that had frustrated them. In his third interview, for example, answering whether or not he had a good relationship with his social worker, Callum said:

> I do, yeah, but the problem with her is she is a bit, I don't know, lazy... she just leaves things to the last minute, like with my flat...sorry about this, we asked her ages before my eighteenth to try and sort out a flat... but she left it until the last minute, and...my provisional driving license, I've got that now, but...it took ages. She is a good social worker but she is very slow at doing things.

A number of designated teachers from non-mainstream schools were outspoken in their criticism of multi-agency working with children's social care, including Mr Grey:

> I mean if we are trying to work together to act as a concerned, well-managed parent, we are not doing the job, because we do not link as a well-managed parent...School does one job, the foster parent does one job...We link together well, very well...and that's on a daily basis... And then social system comes in when they need to come in, to do their admin...It's strong to say it's dysfunctional. I'd say there's a long way to go to get this tight circle around the child.

Social workers: continuity, support and relationships

Some of the problems appeared to derive at least in part from the high turnover of social workers. When asked what she thought was the worst thing about being in care, Devora replied 'them taking their time to do things... so many social workers'. It is frustrating that, despite this issue having been highlighted in the literature repeatedly (Cashmore, 2002; Social Exclusion Unit, 2003; Berridge et al., 2008), it remains a core defect in children's experience of the care system in English-speaking nations (McFadden et al., 2015) and elsewhere, including in Croatia (Sladovic-Franz and Branica, 2013). Social worker continuity was raised repeatedly by young people throughout the CLET study. The quotations below demonstrate the scale of the problem and young people's feelings on the subject:

> I'm not happy about the social worker because the social worker was changing, because like if you stay with the same social worker they understand more about you...in the long-term...they know you very well, and you know them as well, so you know how they work, and they know how you work as well...it's better to have, I would say, like one social worker, and not change (Bashir).
>   I've had about five or six social workers in my care life, and none of them have really worked out...Too many social workers just coming in and out. Just too much. (Callum).

I've had oh so many social workers...in the summer I had a social worker, and then I had another one, and then I have another one, and then she's just said that she's not going to be on my case anymore because she's got a different job in that office...and I'm gonna get another one, so that's just in the space of...six months?...so many social workers. I think it's really bad that, because some children in care are worse off than me, being abused, and they need that one steady thing in their life, and they don't even really get that (Devora).

How many social workers have you had since you've been in care?

I lost count, I don't know. So many (Habib).

I have no idea, they keep on changing... (Imogen).

Can't count...I can't even remember some of their names because they just come and they go, and they come and they go...Half of them I don't remember...They come and go so quickly... (Jacinda).

About seven, eight...In the past year I've had four (Niall).

Designated teachers commented on the difficulties that discontinuity of social workers and stretched social services provision created for interagency working, timely service provision and stability in school:

we worked with a number of boroughs...the social workers from [one] were really good, and really on it, the social workers from [another] were totally overstretched...they were totally disorganised, and often unable to attend meetings, or would cancel meetings. The old story...Social workers would always be changing...and then you'd have to re-establish those relationships again. It was hard to keep track of social workers (Ms Coral).

we struggle...to fill a lot of our social care roles...and it's very difficult to get the calibre of people if you are not willing to value them...I have worked with lots of social workers, some of them are massively brilliant... and some are overwhelmed, or confused, or don't really see, don't get it...sometimes you have to circumnavigate the people you work with to try and get to the core of helping somebody. And it prolongs getting action...and that's very frustrating (Ms Tan).

Mr Black similarly referred to social work retention problems as placing 'a huge amount of pressure on all those trying to support young people'. Mr Brown felt that 'the unsettling effect...on the students can be awful, because they are constantly, constantly, getting a new social worker', while Ms Rose commented that it was much easier when social workers knew their young clients well, so that young people could confide in them, but often that did not seem to be the case.

The direct result of the high social worker turnover, bureaucracy and delays recounted above was that almost all young people described poor relationships with their social workers, although they were generally hesitant to criticize provision and were appreciative of individual support. Bashir, for example, was grateful for the effort his social worker had invested in getting his case for tuition approved through the local authority's panel procedures ('she really worked for it'), while Adam's social worker had 'put in all the effort, I couldn't ask for more off [sic] her really'. Farouk, however, distinguished between the apparent motivation of his current and previous social workers: 'she don't really look supportive…she looks like she's just trying to do her job and that's it, unlike my other social worker, who looked like he kind of wanted to help us'.

When asked whether the staff at her secure unit were supportive, Unity replied:

> Some were and some weren't. I think it's the same as everywhere you go, you get some people that are really doing their job because they want to help you and then some people that are doing it just because it's a job and they don't really actually care.

Frustration at not being listened to could lead to young people disengaging or to active hostility. Tasmin explained why she saw little of her (Polish) social worker:

> I don't turn up because I don't like her…Because I'll ask her stuff and then she just won't get back to you. And then like she's never even in England…

Priya justified her behaviour in terms of forcing social services to take notice:

> It's not really playing up, it's when I say something to social services and they don't listen it's very irritating. So I do stuff that makes them notice, and hear me, because they don't listen when I talk with my mouth, unless I do something with my actions, that's the only time they listen.

It was apparent from their comments that young people were looking for a very different relationship with their social worker than they expected or wanted from educational professionals. Gilroy and Priya were both critical of tutors at their colleges for being 'too young': they felt they were there to learn and needed to be able to respect their tutors, a view echoed by Habib. Gilroy described his experience at college as

> shit…rubbish…couldn't control them, well, couldn't control me especially, I don't know about the others…some listened to him and some didn't. He's too young to be a tutor…just didn't have the thing, just too young.

Priya said she left college because 'the teacher chatted too much basically, she used to sit down and have a conversation with us instead of teaching us, she's quite young'. However, young people's relationships with social workers were much more personal, and understanding, rather than respect, was the most important factor. Qadira said:

> the first one, she didn't know how to talk to me...I probably would be in college by now, but...she didn't know how to persuade me to go...my leaving care social worker, she just knew how to talk to me.

Similarly, Jacinda when asked if any of her social workers stood out, said

> my last one was alright, I just remember her because she was my last one, she was quite young, so she understood, she would talk to me like I was...the same age sort of thing.

Adam was the only one of the group to express regret at a change of social worker as he moved to the leaving care team, attributing this to the longevity of their relationship ('she's been there for me over the years') and his late transfer to the leaving care team to the fact that 'my social worker wanted to keep hold of me'. His new social worker took the trouble to see him monthly to start with 'because he needs to see me more now to find out more about me', in contrast to reports from most young people that social workers made contact according to their administrative agendas, rather than young people's wishes or needs.

Adam's experience was exceptional in this study, however. The high turnover of social workers obviously made it difficult for most young people to form relationships with them, but many felt let down by them. Riley's explanation was typical: 'I just don't get on with social workers...Because they say they'll do something and they don't, or they'll say they'll come and see you and they don't'. Unity had four or five social workers, but said she did not have a good relationship with any, adding

> the one I've got now is the best relationship that I've ever had with a social worker, and that's...we get on, do you know what I mean?...I think...for a lot of years I didn't like them because of my past experience with my first social worker, and that was awful...I don't think she knew her job at all, she didn't have a clue what was best for me...just felt that she didn't do anything to help me, to listen to me...What she wanted to do, was easiest for her, sort of thing.

In her second interview, Kayla was looking forward to developing a relationship with her leaving care social worker. She had seen her only once in the first six months or so since she had been appointed but had recently met her again. They 'decided to meet as frequently as we can' and every six weeks was set down in her review. She described how they would 'go to like the coffee shop and have some hot chocolate and stuff, and just be casual, that was nice...I like her, she's like me, we are both crazy together'. When we met the following year, Kayla was supposed to see her social worker every three months but explained 'now that I'm eighteen it's harder to get in contact with her...so if I text her she might not text me back, or she'll text me back ten days later'. Kayla thought she had enjoyed good relationships with her social workers, but to an extent this appeared to be because her expectations were low. She said 'I think my social workers have all been nice, they wouldn't just abandon us whenever' and that she did not mind the frequent changes. But she added:

> usually I don't like changes, but with social workers I think it's different, I know they are not going to stay for the longest time period as they say they would, so I just get used to it, and say "oh we are getting a new social worker, OK".

These accounts suggest that the high turnover of social work staff and pressured working conditions undermine the potential for effective practice. There has also been growing criticism in England in recent years that the increasingly managerial and process-driven approach to child protection practice has lost sight of the primacy of relationships in social work (Lonne et al., 2009; Munro, 2011). The International Federation of Social Workers' definition of the function of the social work profession has been adopted by the British Association of Social Workers (BASW) (2012: 6) and states:

> The social work profession promotes social change, problem solving in human relationships and the empowerment and liberation of people to enhance well-being. Utilizing theories of human behaviour and social systems, social work intervenes at the points where people interact with their environments.

There was little evidence in this study of such relationship-based practice in young people's accounts of their interactions with the professionals entrusted with their empowerment, but in some cases problems ran deeper than the avoidance of committing to a relationship that was likely to be transient or unreliable. Tasmin, for example, was supposed to be undertaking life story work, but because she had a particularly problematic relationship with her social worker, undertaking such sensitive work was likely to do more harm than good: 'I just want to get rid of her...she gets me really upset and it brings up like anxiety'. Despite her own difficulties with her brother's behaviour, which included stealing from her, she was concerned to protect him from what she saw as poor social work intervention: 'they were just saying oh what they think's best for my brother, and I'm like "no it's not...he's a piece of paper, and your pay cheque, you really don't know him"'. Unity's explanation for her extremely difficult behaviour was 'I just think that I didn't like my social worker, an absolute bitch, I don't think she really thought about how I felt'.

Some young people, such as Habib and Gilroy and the young women in supported housing (Priya, Qadira and Unity), reported better relationships with their key workers than their social workers, but these again appeared to be transient relationships. At 18, Priya, Qadira and Unity would no longer be entitled to the services of the specialist care leavers' charity supporting them. Vulnerable young adults such as Niall would be passed to the transitional team, although all care leavers are now entitled to the support of a personal advisor until age 25 should they request it (Children Act 1989 s23CZB).

Self-reliance, risk and resilience

The cumulative effect of high social work turnover, bureaucratic procedures and delays on young people's engagement with social services tended to manifest in participants taking control over their own lives as far as possible. Many demonstrated considerable initiative in doing so. Often the consequences were positive, but this was more likely in the case of young people who described generally good levels of support from social workers and/or carers. Adam was very appreciative of support from his carers, school and social workers but quick to point out that his success would be down to his own endeavours, coupled with good peer relationships:

> In the beginning I didn't have much support…but I always tried to work hard and whatever I was provided with I'll do what I've got to do…It's nice to have support, but it can still be done, if you've got friends then you can do it…because if I'm not going to do it no one's going to do it for me, are they? You've got to have commitment.

Kayla could have accessed additional support at school in her final year but explained:

> I choose not to because if I get to uni I'm not going to be like "can I have additional support?" Because someone's not gonna be on my back all the time to tell me to catch up, so I'd rather learn to do it myself than have someone do it for me all the time.

Riley said of the inadequate support he received from social workers 'I'm not fussed. I don't think I need it', and that he did not seek assistance from his personal advisor because 'I can do it on my own, don't need them'. The local authority had tried to move him back nearer his home address when he had had to leave the residential care home, but he had refused to go because he knew that he needed to stay away from the people who had led him into trouble in the first place. Bashir and Sofia, both UASC, appeared somewhat self-contained. Bashir chose not to ask for additional help from his carers if he felt it might be 'unfair' to make demands on them, and Sofia stated she had made just one friend at Fairfields, and otherwise she did not talk to anyone. If she had a problem, she said, 'I always have myself'.

Other young people appeared resistant to seeking support because of their experiences. Callum acknowledged that his carer thought that his education was 'very important' and could probably help with issues such as choosing options for the sixth form, but he said 'I just do it all by myself'. Although he had been living with that carer for over four years at the time of the first interview, this attitude is understandable in the context of a placement where he was not happy. Habib had taken to arranging to see his younger siblings himself because his carer was 'not the type of woman' who would arrange it for him. With hindsight, Habib also felt that his expulsion from school was unfair and seemed to suggest that someone should have stood up for him at the time: 'I couldn't defend for myself. I was young and didn't know. If that was me [now] and I could talk for myself...I wouldn't have gone to [the PRU]'. Priya, whose child had seemingly been removed from her care, was more explicit, recounting that 'social services gave me a lot of responsibility after having a child, so I had to do everything for myself, so I did.'

The most vulnerable young people were often those who were most adamant that they controlled decisions in their lives. Gilroy, for example, when asked how much control he felt he had had over decisions in his life stated: 'most of it really...I make my own decisions...if I want to do something I do it'. Qadira stated that she did not listen to her mother, but when asked to whom she did listen she replied: 'I like listening to myself, and doing things in my own way. I don't like listening to no-one'. She explained that she often applied for apprenticeships but didn't attend because she 'couldn't be bothered' or was ill. She elaborated:

> it's just myself. I need to make myself do it. No-one can make me do it, it has to be me...it depends on the way...the outside is going, like with family and stuff like that, with friends...and if I'm happy...then of course I'll attend, but if I'm grumpy and that I won't.

Unity had a similar attitude:

> I think it's all down to myself, whether I want to do it or not, it's all about no one can make you do what you don't want...It's up to yourself, and whether you want to achieve it, put your mind to it.

These young people's accounts resonate with two aspects of the resilience literature: Cameron's concept of self-reliance, and Stein's categorisation of care leavers, in which 'survivors' regard themselves as highly self-reliant, but remain dependent on welfare benefits and social services, and 'strugglers' become alienated from or reject professional support. The following section explores the utility of resilience theory in understanding the trajectories of care leavers as they transition into adulthood.

Resilient adaptation

While the focal model has been used to provide a representation of 'normal' adolescent development which helps to explain the particular challenges faced by children growing up in state care, resilience theory conceptualises how young people at risk of negative life outcomes may nonetheless function well. Resilience is 'a dynamic process wherein individuals display positive adaptation despite experiences of significant adversity or trauma' (Luthar and Cicchetti, 2000: 858). In the context of research with care leavers, a resilience framework can help to explain why some young people do much better than others and what support is most likely to be effective. It is also advantageous in its acknowledgement of children's agency and in facilitating attention to the effects of interaction between the child and their environment, in addition to encouraging a focus on strengths and competence rather than deficits and maladjustment (Luthar and Cicchetti, 2000).

There is a well-developed body of work identifying risk and protective factors in the development of resilient adaptation, from which it appears that while most children and young people recover from short episodes of adversity if protective factors are available, earlier and longer experiences of risk factors are more difficult to overcome (Yates et al., 2003). The relation between these factors and resilience is complex (Coleman, 2011; Zolkoski and Bullock, 2012), however, and it should be borne in mind in the following discussion that the definition and measurement of resilient adaptation remain subject to debate (Zolkoski and Bullock, 2012) and that resilience literature lacks a common cross-disciplinary conceptual framework (Sameroff et al., 2003). Moreover, the resilient adaptation displayed by an individual may vary over time and be exhibited only in some areas of their life (Rutter, 2006) because it develops through the 'steeling' effect (Rutter, 1985: 600) of exposure to manageable levels of adversity. Concepts of risk and resilience cannot be applied to individual young people's experiences in a straightforward way, as critical events and individuals can precipitate unpredictable turns (MacDonald, 2007). Zolkoski and Bullock caution that risk factors are no more than '*probability* statements, the likelihood of a gamble whose levels of risk change depending on the time and place' (2012: 2295).

Specific risk and protective factors pertinent to the care population are considered in the following sections, but some aspects of children's functioning exhibit a more complex relationship with resilient adaptation. Attachment style is one such aspect: secure attachment and resilience appear to share a number of underlying factors and attachment state of mind is a marker of resilience (Gerber, 2007). 'Coping' strategies comprise another (Walsh et al., 2010). The 'coping' literature suggests that people demonstrate different approaches to managing stressors in their lives, which may be adaptive or maladaptive (Coleman, 2011). Survivors of child maltreatment are at risk of higher perceived stress throughout their lives than the general population, which may account for their poorer physical health (e.g. Hager and Runtz, 2012).

Coping strategies are often considered under three categories: problem-focused/active (such as seeking help or rational problem-solving), emotion-focused/internal (including reflection, self-blame and wishful thinking) and avoidance/withdrawal (minimising or denying a problem, delaying address-ing it or seeking distraction) (Seiffge-Krenke, 1995; Hager and Runtz, 2012). Adult victims of child maltreatment display a wide repertoire of coping strategies, both positive and negative: Limke et al. (2010) suggest that they may be able to access the same coping strategies as others in low stress cir-cumstances and that maladaptive strategies may be a particular, and reason-able, response to their individual situations. For example, victims of child sexual abuse appear to be more likely to use avoidant or emotion-focused coping strategies; the former in particular are associated with increased psy-chological distress in adulthood (Walsh et al., 2010).

Age, gender, personality and ethnicity are the most significant correlates of adolescent coping strategies (Frydenberg, 2008). Although it is difficult to tease out differences in coping strategies according to ethnicity because of cultural variations (Coleman, 2011), a study drawing on data from seven European nations found remarkable similarities in coping behaviours over-all (Gelhaar et al., 2007). Adolescents with low self-esteem are more likely to use avoidant strategies (Dumont and Provost, 1999). Older adolescents are more likely to employ distraction strategies, such as drug use and smoking, and have a greater tendency to self-blame than younger ones (Frydenberg, 2008). From around age 15 young people increasingly attempt to communi-cate with the person causing the problem and seek the advice of friends and people experiencing similar issues (Seiffge-Krenke, 1995), although these active coping strategies are utilized more by girls than by boys (Gelhaar et al., 2007). Girls are also more likely to self-harm (Moran et al., 2012), while boys appear more likely to use aggression or confrontational re-sponses (Coleman, 2011).

Risk factors in the lives of children in care

Risk factors are commonly classified into individual, family and community factors, as are the protective factors that have been identified as enabling young people experiencing a high accumulation of risk factors to demon-strate resilient adaptation (Yates et al., 2003; Coleman, 2011; Zolkoski and Bullock, 2012). Individual risk factors include poor health, low intelligence quotient, anxiety, hyperactivity, poor attention and a readiness to become frustrated. Family risk factors include harsh or inconsistent parental dis-cipline; family conflict; parental ill health, involvement in crime, death or divorce; and disruptive siblings. Community factors include poverty, poor housing, poor schooling and high crime rates.

From a resilience perspective, children in care are often highly vulner-able to poor developmental trajectories because of persistent exposure to risk factors from an early age (Coleman and Hagell, 2007) and the inflating effect of cumulative risk factors (Luthar and Cicchetti, 2000). Risk factors are often interconnected in the lives of children in care because of the way in which family and community factors are associated with or impact on individual risk factors. For example, community risk factors such as poverty align with social conditions which create stresses on parenting and thereby increase the conditions in which child maltreatment is more likely, such as harsh or inconsistent discipline or inadequate supervision. Coleman (2011) cites ongoing family conflict and repeated changes of home and school as particular challenges to resilient adaptation in adolescents. These life experiences are perhaps the most common to blight the lives of children in care.

Promoting resilience: protective factors for children in care and care leavers

A number of factors in adolescence can assist the development of resilient adaptation, including a sense of personal agency, good self-concept, a supportive relationship with at least one competent adult, good peer relationships and positive educational experiences (Masten et al., 1990; Luthar and Cicchetti, 2000; Sameroff et al., 2003; Rutter, 2006; Zolkoski and Bullock, 2012). Schools have an important role to play, including through consistent and supportive relationships with staff (Höjer and Johansson, 2013), provision of extracurricular activities (Gilligan, 2000), enabling development of self-esteem and encouraging children's capacity to exercise agency (Schofield, 2001; Rutter, 2006), opportunities for which are often limited in care (Geenen and Powers, 2007; Leeson, 2007). Good school attendance and at least one good friend were the most common protective factors in Honey et al.'s study (2011).

Evidence suggests that girls are more likely to depend on social relationships for support in stressful circumstances (Seiffge-Krenke, 1995), and supportive relationships across a number of domains have been found to be more important for girls than boys (Call and Mortimer, 2001). However, social support is regarded by Coleman as 'critical' (2011: 224), and he concludes that, of all protective factors, for adolescents 'it is the family which plays the key role' (Coleman, 2011: 224). This, coupled with Seiffge-Krenke's finding of the 'great importance of the family in coping with stress' (1995: 226) and that adolescents from conflict-ridden and disengaged families experience high levels of stress but are more likely to withdraw and less likely actively to seek solutions, perhaps contributes to explaining the particular vulnerability of many children in care.

Geenen and Powers (2007) in the US and Schofield (2001) in the UK emphasise the need to maintain caring relationships for children in care through adolescence and into adulthood, but research in both jurisdictions has exposed a dearth of such relationships for many of these children (Geenen and Powers, 2007; Mallon, 2007). Where achieved, these relationships may be found in informal sources, rather than through professionals

(Gilligan, 2008), and as a consequence may be vulnerable to disruption through changes in care arrangements (Driscoll, 2013a). Ahrens et al. (2011) suggest that transition planning for care leavers should formally involve significant non-parental adults; foster youth mentors are carefully matched to young people and receive specialised training; young people are provided with interpersonal skills training; and consideration should be given to instituting mentorship relationships in preparation for times of need.

Coleman (2011: 224) calls for regard to the reciprocity of relationships and 'an emphasis on adolescents as constructors or shapers of their own development'. This is important not least because resilient adaptation in the absence of consistent and caring adult relationships may give rise to an overly strong sense of self-reliance (Dixon et al., 2006; Cameron, 2007; Samuels and Pryce, 2008). Self-reliance may be regarded as an exercise of personal agency and may facilitate the development of the skills required for independence: the young people in Samuel and Pryce's study regarded self-reliance as a positive attribute. However, Cameron (2007) warns of the importance of the context in which self-reliance develops and is exercised, and particularly the role of inadequate support. She suggests that professionals should be wary of regarding care leavers' refusal of professional support as 'difficult' behaviour.

The resilience literature also suggests that the changes in status and functioning associated with transition to adulthood may provide a particular opportunity to redress risk factors from earlier childhood (Masten et al., 2004), a notion referred to in the literature in terms of 'turning points'. Young people leaving care will experience changes in both their personal lives and their education that have the potential to enhance or undermine resilient adaptation. Experience of educational success may act as a 'turning point' by enhancing self-esteem and offering new opportunities (Rutter, 2006; Shepherd et al., 2010) or by engendering a sense of self-efficacy (Drapeau et al., 2007; Hagell, 2007). Development of a relationship of trust with a supportive adult may also initiate a turning point (Drapeau et al., 2007). Accordingly, notwithstanding the importance of stability and continuity in the lives of children in care, the changes associated with leaving care can provide a catalyst for positive change (Dixon et al., 2006; Wade and Munro, 2008). Indeed, despite their generally poor academic and personal outcomes, care leavers often exhibit remarkably resilient adaptation in pursuing their education and career plans in the face of significant practical and emotional challenges (McGloin and Widom, 2001; Allen, 2003; Cameron, 2007; Driscoll, 2013a), although there is some evidence to suggest that young women care leavers are more likely to exhibit resilient adaptation than young men (McGloin and Widom, 2001).

Stein (2006b; 2012: 170) has developed a categorisation of care leavers using a resilience framework, although it is important to bear in mind that resilient adaptation varies over the life course, and the category into which a young person appears to fall should not be regarded as fixed

(Cicchetti, 2013). Stein's revised categories are 'moving on', 'survivors' and 'strugglers' (categorised as 'victims' in Stein's earlier work). Those who are 'moving on' are likely to have benefited from stability, secure attachment and some educational success in care. Most will have left care later than average in a planned move and felt well-prepared for independence, having been able to take advantage of support available to them. They have been able to develop a positive identity through participating in the 'normal' trajectories of further or higher education, partnering and parenthood. 'Survivors' regard themselves as self-reliant, having been shaped by their life circumstances and experiences to be tough and self-sufficient, a view often belied by continuing dependence on services and difficulty in making and keeping supportive relationships. They are likely to have left care younger than those in the 'moving on' group, often in response to a trigger incident such as the breakdown of a foster placement and have limited or no academic qualifications. New supportive relationships, often including less formal ones with personal advisors and/or mentors, may assist this group, as may stable accommodation. Rekindling birth family relationships may be helpful for some, but problematic for others. 'Strugglers' are most at risk of poor life outcomes. They are likely to have experienced the most harmful treatment before entering care, to the extent that the care system is unlikely to achieve stability for them. Cumulative histories of disruption and emotional, psychiatric, behavioural and social problems may culminate in difficulty engaging with and alienation from professional and personal support, leaving care early and a high likelihood of unemployment and homelessness, requiring specialist services.

Combining insights from the theoretical perspectives

Much remains to be understood about the resilient adaptation of maltreated children. The existing research is largely cross-sectional or of limited term if longitudinal and is primarily concerned solely with psychosocial measurements (Cicchetti, 2013). There is considerable congruity between findings from research drawing on attachment theory, coping strategies and resilience, particularly in relation to the importance of consistent supportive relationships. It also appears that although secure attachment may provide a significant opening for resilient adaptation, there may be scope for the development of coping skills to compensate for attachment difficulties: for example, Limke et al. (2010) found that some emotionally or sexually abused individuals with anxious attachment styles were able to use avoidant coping strategies to minimise their exposure to distressing situations. The coping literature is of practical benefit because of its implications for targeted support. While many of the personal and family risk factors from the resilience literature are not amenable to change, young people's coping skills can be utilized and enhanced to promote their resilience through, for example, access to supportive adults and promotion of their sense of agency and self-concept.

Attention to the developmental tasks of adolescence reinforces the importance of attention to relationships in the promotion of resilient adaptation in adolescents. The proposal in Coleman's (1974) focal model of adolescence that adolescents address one issue at a time may contribute to explaining the unpredictability of resilient adaption and the way in which young people's vulnerability to risk factors may vary according to time and place and their reaction to critical events or people in their lives (MacDonald, 2007; Zolkoski and Bullock, 2012). The focal model is also central to consideration of the resilient adaptation of adolescents because it starts from an understanding of adolescents as shapers of their own development. For young people brought up in state care, this work will be constrained by many factors, including the effect of their attachment style on self-worth and the many stressors and risk factors in their lives. In addition, their capacity to develop and to exercise agency is limited compared with that of peers growing up in their birth families. When seen in the context of the focal model, with its emphasis on adolescents as active in their own development and the centrality of relational tasks in adolescent development, the self-reliance of young people who have experienced a dearth of consistent caring relationships in their lives before and in care seems almost inevitable.

Superficially, it may be tempting to regard care leavers' exhibition of self-reliance as evidence of the exercise of autonomy. But Stein's classification of care leavers according to their resilient adaptation, endorsed by the data from the CLET study, demonstrates that the most vulnerable young people – that is, those most in need of continuing support from the state – are likely to demonstrate the most determined self-reliance. These young people are consequently likely to be denied, or to choose to deny themselves, the professional and relational support they need to achieve the skills and conditions for 'full' autonomy, which, it will be recalled, incorporates the notion of autonomy as a relational concept (Hollingsworth, 2013b). Such a conceptualization allows for attention to be paid to the way in which young people's developing identities are shaped by their relationships and social experiences and to how the choices available to young people and the way in which they exercise them are influenced by the interaction between young people and their social worlds. In her identification of 'foundational' rights, Hollingsworth (2013b) stresses the significance of the *quality* rather than merely the *form* of young people's relationships: the importance of this distinction is abundantly clear from the data and discussion in this chapter.

This chapter has considered in depth the many challenges faced by the state in carrying out its parental role for young people in care in the arena of their personal lives and relationships. The evidence base from attachment theory, the focal model, coping strategies and resilience emphasises the enormous significance of relationships and social support in adolescence. From this and the preceding chapter, it is clear that many children and young people in care experience indefensible deficiencies in the level of care they receive in these domains of their lives. Yet it is also evident that many of the factors pertinent to resilient adaptation are not easily amenable to intervention, not least because of the relationship between maltreatment and risk factors for resilience and the tendency for risk factors to cluster and be interrelated. Moreover, personal relationships are not predictable, so that however well-matched a child might appear to be to their carer, social worker or key worker, there is never a guarantee that a child will be able to draw on that relationship for support, perhaps particularly in the case of adolescents, and certainly when self-reliance is entrenched.

Positive educational experiences are also important in the development of resilient adaptation, and educational success may provide a 'turning-point'. While this and the previous chapter have demonstrated the inextricably linked relationship between children's care and their education, academic achievement has been identified as a key factor in determining adult well-being in relation to fostered children in the US (Pecora et al., 2006) and children brought up in care in the UK (Jackson and Martin, 1998). Evidence from Sweden supports Sonia Jackson's claim that low educational attainment is the most concerning risk factor for poor outcomes experienced by children in state care (Berlin et al., 2011). School can provide a stable environment where children do not need to feel 'different'. Educational provision which will enable children to exercise rational decision-making and engage in political and community life is also a 'foundational' right identified by Hollingsworth (2013b). The following chapters consider the importance of education to the life prospects of children brought up in state care and examine how the existing 'attainment gap' might be addressed as they transition out of care.

5 Education, care and life chances

The importance of education: from the personal to the global

Education and 'well-being'

In an essay exploring evidence of the influence of education on happiness and/or well-being, Michalos (2008) provides a lengthy list of the identified benefits of educational attainment, including reference to education as: the main source of human capital, which drives the production of new knowledge and ideas; predictive of economic growth at national level; influential in determinants of health status and healthy lifestyles, including maintenance of a healthy weight; protective against incarceration for criminal offences; predictive of increased longevity; and associated with higher rates of employment as well as access to better paid and more secure employment. In particular, university graduates enjoy higher status and better paid jobs than non-graduates (Lee, 2014; OECD, 2015). Higher educational qualifications are also associated with a greater sense of political efficacy, higher likelihood of volunteer work and greater interpersonal trust. Although all these factors might be expected to be influential in relation to life satisfaction, there is a substantial body of work suggesting that people's level of educational attainment has only a small *direct* effect on their subjective well-being as adults (Michalos, 2008). These issues touch upon the wider literature on the 'economics of happiness', which cannot be covered here but which confirms the importance of employment status (and particularly unemployment) for (un)happiness (Clark, 2003) and a complex but significant relationship at the individual level between income (particularly relative income) and happiness (Graham and Felton, 2006; Clark et al., 2008).

The literature in this area predominantly applies the terms happiness, life satisfaction and subjective well-being to concepts of abstract or felt life outcomes, often interchangeably (Graham and Felton, 2006), although critics point out that well-being is a broader concept than happiness, which tends to be limited to extended sensations of pleasure or good mood, and that subjective measures of what constitutes a good life are necessary but not sufficient (Michalos, 2008). Despite difficulties in the conceptualisation and measurement of well-being and happiness, the concepts are important because measurements of 'successful' outcomes in adulthood that rely on purely economic indicators do not adequately capture people's satisfaction with their lives. For example, in the long-term, there is no relationship between national economic growth and life satisfaction in either developed or less developed nations (Easterlin et al., 2010), and while there is a generally negative relationship between inequality and happiness, this effect varies across groups in different national contexts, possibly partially dependent upon whether inequality is regarded as indicative of social mobility and opportunity or as a marker of persistent disadvantage (Graham and Felton, 2006).

Michalos surmises that although educational attainment may not be particularly influential in relation to the subjective well-being of most groups of people in most domains of their lives, it may have particular impact for some groups. In addition to US and UK studies identifying the significance of academic achievement to the success and well-being of adults from a care background (Jackson and Martin, 1998; Pecora et al., 2006), a Swedish study based on population-level data found low educational attainment to be an important predictor of psychosocial difficulties in adulthood for young people who have been in long term care (Berlin et al., 2011). The reasons for this finding are unclear, but the following sections consider two areas in which research on the significance of educational attainment has focused: self-esteem and social mobility.

Education and self-esteem

Much of the literature on self-esteem in the context of schooling presupposes that self-esteem predicts educational success, although the relationship appears to be reciprocal (de Araujo and Lagos, 2013). Although there is an association between high *general* self-esteem and academic attainment, it has not been found to be large in some studies, and generic programmes to boost self-worth have generally shown little impact on academic attainment (Pullmann and Allik, 2008). Moreover, the association itself is not consistent across groups. In a study drawing on a nationally representative sample of over 4,500 Estonian school children, Pullmann and Allik (2008) found that amongst more academically able students, lower general self-esteem was associated with slightly higher grades, perhaps attributable to more critical self-appraisal. Academic self-esteem was a much better predictor of school achievement.

Self-esteem appears to be a more important factor in educational attainment for boys than for girls (de Araujo and Lagos, 2013). Children of Asian heritage are likely to do better in US schools than their peers, despite low self-esteem, while Black students tend to have high self-esteem but perform relatively poorly (Bankston and Zhou, 2002). Bankston and Zhou conclude that variations in school performance according to racial or ethnic categorisation are not attributable to differences in self-esteem, but, rather, self-esteem appears slightly to ameliorate racial trends in school attainment. Honey et al. (2011) found children in care to have similarly higher self-esteem and general self-perceptions than their peers. First and second generation immigrant children in US schools are more likely to suffer from low self-esteem but generally do well at school, an apparent paradox possibly accounted for by parental drive for upward social mobility (Bankston and Zhou, 2002).

Self-esteem in adulthood is significantly determined by educational attainment (de Araujo and Lagos, 2013), and the relationship between self-esteem in adolescence and wages in adulthood appears to be mediated to a considerable degree by education (Girtz, 2014). These findings add weight to Berlin et al.'s (2011) conclusion that investment in the education of children in care and beyond should be a primary policy focus.

Education and social mobility

One area in which the benefits of educational attainment have been particularly contested relates to social mobility. Predictors of adult social status remain poorly understood, in spite of a considerable research base on the issue (von Stumm et al., 2010). In particular, there is conflicting evidence as to the impact of education on upward social mobility (Breen, 2010; Scherger and Savage, 2010). The 20th century saw an enormous rise in the attainment of formal educational qualifications in developed nations (Breen, 2010), accompanied by a general trend of upward mobility. There is a strong positive correlation between educational attainment and socioeconomic success (de Araujo and Lagos, 2013): OECD data demonstrates that earnings have risen with the level of education attained in all nations for which statistics are available (OECD, 2015) and that the discrepancy in earnings by education qualifications increases with age. At first glance, therefore, the assumption of policy-makers that education is key to enhancing social mobility seems unassailable. In recent years, education policy reform in the UK from both sides of the political divide, and in particular the requirement that young people remain in education and/or training until the age of 18, has been justified in terms of the aim of enhancing social mobility (Sturgis and Buscha, 2015). Yet the available evidence is problematic in a number of ways, including the existence of conflicting evidence as to trends in social mobility. Measurement of absolute social mobility does not in itself indicate that class barriers to advancement have been overcome: instead, studies often use a measure of 'relative' social mobility in order to identify movement by individuals between different social class groups after accounting for generic mobility trends. Additionally, educational attainment varies according to ethnicity in a way which often reinforces social class divisions. For example, differences in socioeconomic status, including the prevalence of single-parenthood, account for the gap in academic attainment between

Black and White American adolescents to a significant degree (Bankston and Zhou, 2002).

A well-respected body of research suggests that social class in midlife is partially predicted by educational attainment, childhood intelligence (IQ), behaviour difficulties and social class of origin (von Stumm et al., 2010; Forrest et al., 2011). All such studies share ambiguities such as the extent to which IQ reflects 'raw' ability or social origins, even where educational experiences are taken into account, and whether socioeconomic status is entirely a reflection of unearned privilege; however, from an analysis of three generations of Scottish men derived from two data sets, Johnson et al. (2010: 64) conclude that the data supports the contention that 'education is the fundamental mechanism acting both to hold individuals in the social class to which they were born and to make possible their movement from one class to another'.

Goldthorpe (2016) disagrees, arguing that education acts as no more than a *positional* good – that is, it is an individual's educational status relative to their competitors in the labour market, rather than in absolute terms, that is significant. He points to the fact that the upward social mobility of the 20th century mostly benefited a group with limited educational qualifications. Goldthorpe reaches two important conclusions: first, that education has limited power to affect overall social mobility but acts only to determine which individuals achieve social mobility, and second, that it is parents' ability to support their children in education and into work that perpetuates the status of families in more advantaged classes. Endorsing this second point in a commentary on neoliberal policies in Australia which encourage students to take responsibility for their own career planning, Billett et al. (2010) point out that in the complexities of modern transitions to adulthood – Arnett's (2000) 'emerging adulthood' – parental social, cultural and economic capital are highly influential in the successful negotiation of these transitions (and see Atkins (2016) in relation to the UK). Consequently, the risks inherent in modern individualized and uncertain transitions are borne disproportionately by young people lacking such family resources.

The critical role of social, political and economic contexts in shaping patterns of social mobility is also discussed by Putnam (2015), who argues convincingly from his research with young people and their parents that as inequality has widened in the US in recent years, consequent upon neoliberal economic policies, it has become increasingly difficult for poor young people to escape the disadvantage of their childhoods. This is very likely to be the case in the UK too, where Goldthorpe (2016: 95) finds that – contrary to much popular commentary – there is no overall decline in social mobility, but the upward social mobility trend seen in the 20th century is reversing, a situation he concludes 'could have far-reaching socio-political consequences', as young people are starting out from a position of relatively high social class and are more likely to experience downward mobility.

Consequently, as the CLET participants and their peers transition into independent adulthood they face both gaping inequality and a downward social mobility trend, a situation in which it appears that parental endeavour is critical to their life chances. It is clear in this context that the corporate parent cannot abdicate responsibility for young people's transitions to work if care leavers are to have any chance of equal opportunity. Social workers in the UK have in the past tended to be reluctant to engage in what some re-garded as social engineering, but in more recent years there has been greater attention to career planning, including at local authority (corporate parent) level. Wadebridge, for example, was implementing a 'Care to Work' plan at the time of the CLET study, which provided young people with work expe-rience placements and apprenticeships and developed employability skills, targeted primarily at low-achieving children.

The changing nature of young people's career prospects complicates the picture set out above. The following section explores the related con-cerns that: first, while a more educated workforce may not in the past have fuelled upward social mobility, it might be necessary to avoid further downward movement; and second, that higher educational attainment may be necessary to access opportunities in a globalised and technologically-advanced job market.

Meeting the skills needs of technologically-advanced nations

Globalisation and the rise of the technological society have significantly altered the skills sets required by employees in a rapidly-changing environ-ment where complex problems may emerge in new contexts (Greiff et al., 2014). Across OECD countries, employment rates are generally higher for people with higher levels of education: average employment rates are around 83 per cent for graduates but only 56 per cent for those who have not completed upper secondary education,[1] for example (OECD, 2015). For governments, the benefits of public investment in education through reduced social welfare costs and increased tax returns exceed the costs; consequently, recent years have seen pre-primary and upper secondary education become universal in most countries (Hodgen et al., 2013; OECD, 2015). In England, young people are now required to remain in education and/or training until they are 18 (Education and Skills Act 2008; Educa-tion Act 2011).

Enrolment in tertiary education has expanded rapidly across the globe in the last half century. Increased enrolment appears to enable economic development, as well as having the potential to open opportunities beyond the societal elite (Yu and Delaney, 2016). Since the increase in graduates has not led to a decline in the average returns on higher education, the OECD concludes that there is no risk of a glut of graduates (OECD, 2014). Rather, it reports concerns that the supply of skilled employees is at risk of failing to keep up with the need for an appropriately skilled workforce in a rapidly changing world. It also suggests that public investment in education may be an appropriate strategy in economic downturns, through reducing unemployment while concurrently developing the national skills base. However, the OECD acknowledges some mismatch between the skills of new graduates and those required by employers (in particular a dearth of science and engineering graduates), leading to a recent increase in graduates in formerly 'non-graduate' occupations in the aftermath of the global recession (OECD, 2014) and more precarious career pathways for some graduates. Concurrently, despite supranational and national rhetoric, developed economies have seen an increase in short-term, insecure and poorly-paid employment, coinciding in neoliberal economies with reduced welfare and social service provision (Billett et al., 2010).

For non-graduates, in most OECD countries vocational upper secondary or post-secondary qualifications and ICT skills provide better employment opportunities than general qualifications, an outcome attributed by the OECD to the development of high-quality vocational education and training (VET) programmes in some countries (OECD, 2015). However, while Germany and Singapore have developed relatively high status VET systems, in both these countries students are diverted into academic or vocational pathways at the beginning of secondary education (Hodgen et al., 2013). In England, the Wolf Review (Wolf, 2011: 11) highlighted the importance of ensuring that young people are not 'tracked in irreversible ways' even before they reach 16, a concern of particular pertinence in relation to young people with disrupted personal and educational histories whose full academic potential may not yet be evident. However, it is a more general issue at a time when there is a sharp divide between the prospects of young people taking academic as opposed to vocational or skills-based qualifications. In England, young people aged 14–19 in vocational or skills-based programmes predominantly come from low socioeconomic backgrounds and have poor school attainment; they are likely to face an extended school-to-work transition and, notwithstanding government rhetoric, precarious, poorly-paid and low-skilled work (Atkins, 2010, 2016). In a broader international context, as the qualifications required for high-status employment increase, young people with lower qualifications face constrained and uncertain futures (Billett et al., 2010).

The government has attempted to respond to this situation in England after the Wolf Review found a lack of high quality vocational qualifications and pathways for young people aged 14–19, coupled with a tendency for educational accountability measures to encourage young people to opt for easier courses, associated with limited prospects, at a cost to basic skills in mathematics and literacy (Wolf, 2011). Students who have not attained Maths and English GCSE at grades A*-C are now required to continue studying these subjects in their 16–19 programme or apprenticeship. The 'apprenticeship offer' under the Education Act 2011 s69 is open not only to all young people aged 16 to 18 but also care leavers aged 19 to 24, giving recognition to the delayed progress of many such young people (Apprenticeships, Skills, Children and Learning Act 2009 s83A(5)).

These extended opportunities for young people to acquire basic skills must be contextualised with reference to the inequitable and divergent opportunities available to young people considered above, as well as to critiques of neoliberal economic policies as promoting VET 'primarily as a source of "work ready" human capital' in response to the perceived needs of a globalised economy rather than a first step on a career path and the promotion of social justice (Atkins, 2016: 5). Nonetheless, they may improve the prospects of some young people in England, including care leavers (although most were not in force at the time of the CLET study). This is crucial in light of the difficulties children in care face in achieving academic qualifications in the timescales imposed by formal educational systems, an issue discussed after brief consideration of study participants' attitudes to education.

The importance of education in the eyes of the research cohort

Despite the difficulties in coping with the demands of school life outlined in Chapter 3, without exception the young people in the CLET study acknowledged the importance of education, and particularly qualifications, for their future success. This is in keeping with English studies such as that of Ball et al. (2000) in relation to young people more generally, but in contrast to the findings of Allen (2003) that care leavers came to value education and training late, through bitter experience of the job market. It accords however with findings from the YiPPEE study, in which young people regarded education as central to moving on from the difficulties of their childhood backgrounds (Johansson and Höjer, 2012; Bryderup and Trentel, 2013; Monserrat et al., 2013), and a study from Croatia (Sladovic-Franz and Branica, 2013). On the whole, previous concerns apparent from the literature of low expectations of children in care and prioritization of practical independence skills over longer-term career goals by professionals (SEU, 2003; Berridge, 2007), appeared to have been replaced by the same pressure to achieve reported to be experienced by this generation more generally (e.g. MindFull, 2013).

The high priority accorded to their education by most of the young people in the CLET study was reflected in the fact that the most common response given to questions about current priorities in their life related to their education, for example:

> *What would you describe as your key priorities in life now?*
> Focusing on college, and...focusing on college (Habib).

Even those young people not in education, employment or training recognized the value of education: Priya, for example, commented that education 'is a good thing'. Priya had entered care when pregnant at the age of 13 and had experienced foster care and four care homes before obtaining her own (supported) accommodation. She had left school at 16 and had dropped out of college after less than a term. Although she had applied for some apprenticeships and jobs, she had tended to fail to turn up for interviews or trial periods. Priya's ready acceptance of education as a social good is highlighted here because she provides a poignant case study of a young person who falls into Stein's category of 'strugglers' (Stein, 2012). Despite an acute difficulty in engaging with professionals and others, arising directly from her personal history, she expressed a clear appreciation of the importance of qualifications.

Unity had spent time in a secure children's home. Although she found the environment oppressive ('I hated being locked in, getting locked in your bedroom, you know what I mean? You can't go out nowhere, it's awful'), she appreciated the enforced education:

> it was a normal school structured day from nine till three, so you'd be doing the normal lessons you would be doing in school, so that was one of the best things I think about the secure unit, a really good school.

Participants were asked whether, if they could go back in time, they would change anything in relation to their education. Around half raised the kind of issues that would be common for this age group, such as choice of subjects, but often the responses related to behaviour and focus, for example:

> I would have stopped bunking...I slapped a teacher, which I regret, got into loads of fights, bunked a lot of lessons (Callum).
> I wish I'd behaved a bit more and done my homework. Done the class work, and then I'd probably get higher than what I am now (Tasmin).
> Go back to school...and when I went to [PRU] I would not have messed around in school (Habib).

Five of the participants (Habib, Niall, Qadira, Riley and Unity) had been in a Pupil Referral Unit (PRU) and Luis was in a school for children with social, educational and behavioural difficulties. All six of these young people expressed the wish that they had focused and behaved better at school – or had been able to do so – or at least had managed to stay in school. For example:

> ...*would you do anything differently?*
> Yeah, of course, I'd go to school. Sometimes when I see kids in their uniform I'm like "oh I wish I could go back to school like that" (Qadira).
> *Is there anything you'd change?*
> My behaviour, and actually turn up on time, stay in school, listen, get my work done. Do all that (Riley).

Those with behavioural problems that had affected their education demonstrated insight into the loss and frustration over barriers to their access to education:

> when I was younger I done bad stuff, and I wasn't good at school, and I was losing my education for a bit of fun....when I'm older, and I'm leaving school, and I've got no education, it's not going to be funny then (Niall).
>
> probably try and stay in education as long as I can...Because I didn't do my GCSEs, because I was in a classroom that was non-GCSE because they didn't think I'd make it...Now this year I stayed on because I wanted to take them, and I did (Luis).

The educational attainment of children in state care

The attainment 'gap'

Notwithstanding the fact that young people valued education, the quotations above demonstrate that they struggled to put good intentions into practice, and their qualifications at the age of 16 reflected that, as well as the educational deficits and other challenges they brought with them into care. Table 5.1 shows the young people's attainment at GCSE and their destinations thereafter. The table shows that of the 19 young people whose qualifications are known, only four attained 5A*-Cs at GCSE at age 16, including Maths and English (the government's benchmark at the time), but at least a further three, Adam, Imogen and Kayla, did so through repeating courses the following year.

The low educational attainment of children in care compared to all children has been a matter of concern internationally for some years (Stein, 2008; Pecora, 2012; Font and Maguire-Jack, 2013). A systematic review of 28 studies published in English after 1990 (27 of which came from the US, Australia, Canada and the UK) (O'Higgins et al., 2015) found that internationally, children in state care perform less well than their peers in school grades, literacy and numeracy scores, attendance rates and school exclusion. The YiPPEE project found a similar pattern of underachievement in all five of the participating European countries (Denmark, Hungary, Spain, Sweden and the UK) (Cameron et al., 2012; Johansson and Höjer, 2012). Authors of the Spanish study describe the attainment of children in care as 'far below' that of their peers, even for those who have spent many years in care (Monserrat et al., 2013: 13). Analysis of Swedish population data for children born between 1972 and 1981 showed 27 per cent of graduates from long-term foster care received no post-16 education, compared with six per cent of the population in general and 22 per cent of children who received social service support while remaining at home (Berlin et al., 2011). In Denmark, around 16 per cent of care leavers do not complete compulsory school compared with six per cent of their peers (Bryderup and

Table 5.1 Young people's attainment and destinations

Name	Qualifications at 16	School/college 16+
5 A*-C inc. Maths & English at 16		
Bashir	4 A*s, 8 As, 1 B (English)	School
Devora	2 As, 7 Bs, 1 C, 1 pass, 1 D	College (Performing Arts)
Jacinda	2Bs; 4Cs (2 English, Maths, Science); 1 Merit; 1D, 1E	School then repeated Year 12 in College
Tasmin	Media, sociology, business, history, core subjects	School
5 A*-C inc. Maths & English 16+		
Adam	6/7 A*s at GCSE, Maths resit	School
Imogen	2 Ds, 3 Es, 2 Fs, 1G	College (Child care)
Kayla	Ds in English and Maths,	School
Sofia?	Took Maths, English, Science, Dance GCSEs	College
Did not achieve 5 A*-C		
Callum	'a couple of passes.'	School
Farouk	'Most everything Ds'	College (immigration exclusion)
Gilroy	[grades not stated]	College (excluded for behavior)
Habib	Limited GCSE courses at PRU, qualifications unclear	College (level 1)
Luis	No qualifications Year 11, expecting Ds/Es Year 12	Repeated Year 11 in SEBD special school then College
Niall	Functional skills & 2 GCSEs in Year 11	College (excluded)
Ollie	None	Will be dependent throughout life
Priya	? no quals / some BTECs	College (dropped out)
Qadira	NVQ level 1 in hair & literacy	Neither – left school Year 10
Riley	Ds, Es and Fs	College (dropped out)
Unity	Limited secondary attend'ce	College (dropped out)
Qual status unclear		
Elliott	Coursework 'mostly Bs & Cs'	College (dropped out first term)
Michael	Qualifications unknown	School

Trentel, 2013); in Israel, only about 40 per cent of care leavers graduate from high school (Sulimani-Aidan, 2015). German care leavers have high levels of school refusal and are more likely to leave school early than their peers (Zeller and Köngeter, 2012), while young people in care in Hungary are more likely to be in vocational-pathway or remedial schools than their peers (Rácz and Korintus, 2013). Children in care in the US perform below grade level, are at greater risk of having to repeat a grade and are less likely to graduate from high school or attend college, while experiencing higher rates of suspension or expulsion and placement in special education (Trout et al., 2008; Font and Maguire-Jack, 2013). The general population pattern of superior academic attainment by girls compared with boys in Western nations is reflected in the care population (Kirk et al., 2012; Flynn et al., 2013; Romano et al., 2015).

In some developed nations, there remain inadequate data and attention to the school attendance, participation and achievement of children in care, including the Republic of Ireland (Darmody et al., 2013), Canada (Ferguson and Wolkow, 2012) and Croatia (Sladović-Franz and Branica, 2013). In the UK, systematic data have been collected at the national level since 1999 and policy directly targeting this issue date from the *Quality Protects* initiative in 1998 (Berridge et al., 2008). In England, in the year ending 31st March 2016, 58.8 per cent of all children in the relevant age cohort achieved A*-C in Maths and English, but only 17.5 per cent of children in care (DfE/NS, 2017). Boys perform particularly poorly, as do children with a high score in the Strengths and Difficulties Questionnaire (SDQ),[2] but the wide disparity in attainment between this cohort and their peers diminishes considerably if special educational needs are taken into consideration (Sebba et al., 2015). Although changes in data collection methods render comparisons with previous years difficult, overall there is evidence of a slight narrowing of the attainment gap in the last few years. The following section considers the complexity of the reasons for the differential between children in care and their peers and the extent to which care systems do or can improve educational outcomes for children of the state.

Understanding the attainment gap

Children's entry into care generally results from a range of factors in themselves associated with low educational attainment (Berridge et al., 2008; Hannon et al., 2010); consequently, many enter care with cognitive deficits relative to their peers (Stone, 2007). The diversity of the care population is such that the underlying causes of children's educational difficulties are many and challenging, and possible genetic explanations should not be discounted (Rutter, 2000). In addition to the higher incidence of mental health problems and special educational needs in this population, children commonly come from backgrounds of socioeconomic disadvantage (Stone, 2007; Berridge, 2012; Cameron et al., 2012). There is a wealth of research evidence on the association between low socioeconomic status and poor educational attainment and some evidence that the relationship is a causal one (Blandon and Gregg, 2004). Childhood maltreatment itself is robustly associated with poor literacy, mathematical skills and school attendance, independently of sociodemographic factors associated with maltreatment such as poverty (Stone, 2007). Although there is a limited evidence base as to the causal mechanisms by which maltreatment affects educational attainment in the longer term (Slade and Wissow, 2007), the literature highlights the twin pathways of poor academic skills and behavioural difficulties. US research suggests that there is some differentiation of academic problems by type of maltreatment experienced, with neglect being particularly associated with poor academic skills and physical abuse with behavioural difficulties in school (Stone, 2007; Romano et al., 2015). Greater intensity of maltreatment (measured by factors including frequency, subtype and exposure to multiple subtypes of maltreatment) and exposure to initial maltreatment at an earlier age are associated with poorer academic performance (Slade and Wissow, 2007; Romano et al., 2015). Behavioural difficulties and grade retention are particularly likely where there has been maltreatment at an early age (Stone, 2007).

There is now recognition that both children's pre-care and in-care experiences must be taken into consideration in evaluating young people's educational outcomes (Stone, 2007; O'Higgins et al., 2015). In England and North America, the attainment gap is greater for older children than it is in lower year groups (DfE/NS, 2017; Romano et al., 2015), but at least in the English context, this in itself should not be regarded as necessarily reflecting a failure in the care system. Rather, due to the transitory nature of children's encounters with care, coupled with many children's late entry into care, older school children comprise a rather different cohort than those in lower year groups. For example, most UASC will enter care over the age of 14. Although they are often highly motivated and make good progress (Jackson et al., 2005; Cameron et al., 2012), many start school in this country with little English and limited prior education. Other explanations may include problems often exhibited by adolescent entrants into care and the fact that less troubled younger children may leave the care system through adoption, special guardianship or return to their birth families (Sebba et al., 2015). Moreover, in the English context, educational outcomes for children entering care over age 10 are better for those who spend longer in care (Sebba et al., 2015), provided that their experience is relatively stable in terms of placement and school changes and returns to their family of origin.

While the picture is complex, O'Higgins et al. (2015) found little evidence from their international systematic review that care itself is damaging to children's educational attainment, but neither did it appear to provide educational benefits. Font and Maguire-Jack (2013) in the US are less confident, concluding that it is still not clear whether care itself or children's associated circumstances and previous maltreatment are primarily responsible for the poor achievement of this cohort. Certainly to date, public care systems have not enabled most children to make up the deficit arising from their earlier experiences, either in Europe (Höjer et al., 2008) or the US (Pecora, 2012), although there is limited research on the academic trajectories of children in care in some countries, including Germany (Zeller and Köngeter, 2012) and Spain (Monserrat et al., 2013). Unless research takes into account pre-existing factors affecting educational attainment, such as socioeconomic status and learning difficulties (much does not), the effects of pre-care experiences and of care intervention cannot be disentangled (Stone, 2007). For some groups, such as indigenous Australian youth, there may be compounding historical and cultural factors that render enabling educational aspiration and attainment particularly challenging (Harvey et al., 2016). With this context in mind, the remainder of this section discusses the evidence base in relation to in-care factors associated with children's educational outcomes, particularly placement type and stability, support from professionals and carers and children's unmet emotional and mental health needs.

It is difficult to assess the effect of placement type on educational achievement. For example, although young people in kinship and foster placements gained better results than those in residential accommodation in Flynn et al.'s study (2013), this appeared to be accounted for almost entirely by the characteristics of children placed in residential care. Contrary to the weight of previous literature, Font's (2014) study involving 1,215 children in kinship or foster care found kinship care to be negatively associated with reading scores and did not find improved behaviour effects, particularly for children with poorer functioning upon entry, but these findings may be attributable to the financial and social disadvantages widely faced by kinship carers compared with foster carers, which often include lower educational attainment and less training.

Placement instability, including multiple attempts at rehabilitation home and associated changes of school, has been identified internationally as particularly damaging to children's educational prospects (SEU, 2003; Allen and Vacca, 2010; Pecora, 2012; Bryderup and Trentel, 2013; Sebba et al., 2015). The effect of placement stability on school changes and attendance is particularly concerning (Zorc et al., 2013; Pears et al., 2015), and Pecora (2012) highlights the additional stigma attaching to children who are held back a grade, a common experience for children in care in the US (Stone, 2007). Bottrell (2009) asserts that resistance to participation in normative activities such as education may represent, from the young person's perspective, protective adaptation, through rejection of discourses which construct them as of little worth.

Research also highlights the importance of having encouraging adults for young people's educational success (e.g. Monserrat et al., 2013). Poor educational attainment has been blamed in part on teachers' low expectations of children in England in the past (SEU, 2003) and has been identified more recently elsewhere: see for example Sladović-Franz and Branica (2013) in relation to Croatia. The role of teachers appeared to be more significant than that of carers in determining educational success in Sebba et al.'s (2015) English study, but early support for education in birth families was often a feature in the lives of educationally successful young people. Low priority being accorded to their education by social workers and carers has been identified as detrimental to young people's success in European research (Jackson and Cameron, 2012). Limited engagement in young people's education by foster carers has also been identified as a concern in some US and Canadian research (O'Brien, 2012; Weinberg et al., 2014). While carers' educational aspirations for the child are predictive of academic attainment (Flynn et al., 2013; Harvey et al., 2016), English and Australian carers have often been found to be poorly equipped to offer academic support (Berridge, 2007; Harvey et al., 2016). A Canadian study of approaching 700 children in Ontario aged 10–15 found academic achievement to be associated with caregivers who provided high academic expectations; access to books; and home-based academic support, but no significant association between caregivers' school-based involvement and higher attainment (Cheung et al., 2012). Low assessments of young people's potential coupled with pressure to prepare for independent living still combine to steer care leavers into vocational pathways (Rácz and Korintus, 2013; Sladovic-Franz and Branica, 2013).

The significance of a consistent and caring adult advocate for children's achievement has emerged from research in the US care system (Pecora, 2012), as well as in Germany (Albus et al., 2010, cited in Zeller and Köngeter, 2012) and Denmark (Bryderup and Trentel, 2013). Sebba et al.'s interviews with 26 English young people revealed that their life 'needed to matter to others before it could matter to them' (2015: 6) and the importance of people they could trust not to let them down and whom reciprocally they did not want to let down. Consistent with the tendency for this group to exhibit high levels of self-reliance, young people in Sebba et al.'s study were likely to regard their educational progress as 'down to them' (2015: 6) (see also Bryderup and Trentel, 2013 and Sladovic-Franz and Branica, 2013), but the research pointed to the importance of children being emotionally ready to accept adult support. Continuing difficulties with birth family members could undermine efforts to promote young people's progress at school.

Children's mental health and emotional needs can also significantly affect their performance in school (Association of Directors of Children's Services/National Consortium for Examination Results/National Association of Virtual School Heads, 2015; Pecora, 2012). Behavioural difficulties are particularly associated with poorer outcomes (Flynn et al., 2013). Exclusion and absence from school, particularly unauthorised absence, are strongly predictive of poorer GCSE performance (Sebba et al., 2015). Although there is little research which directly considers the relationship between children's academic attainment and their mental health, the association appears to be bidirectional (Romano et al., 2015). Educational progress is affected in accordance with the severity of young people's emotional and behavioural difficulties (Biehal et al., 2009), but insufficient attention is paid to children's emotional, mental and physical health needs (Blower et al., 2004; Ford et al., 2007; Noonan et al., 2012). In a review of the literature, Welbourne and Leeson (2013) conclude that the provision of additional educational support is only likely to benefit children significantly if combined with appropriate therapeutic support, including specialist assessment of children's educational needs.

Engagement in further and higher education

Some highly motivated care leavers have accessed, and succeeded in, higher education (Ajayi and Quigley, 2006; Stein, 2008), but for the vast majority, university remains out of reach. Some modest progress appears to have been made in England following the introduction of leaving care services, but only eight per cent of care leavers were in higher education at the age of 21 in 2016 (DfE/NS, 2016a), compared with an initial higher education participation rate of 48 per cent for 17–30 year-olds in 2014–15 (DfE/NS, 2016c). Surprisingly little is known about care leavers' participation in further and higher education in Europe as a whole (Jackson and Cameron, 2010), but the findings of the YiPPEE project confirm that there are similar barriers to higher education for young people ageing out of state care elsewhere in Europe (Cameron et al., 2012). In Denmark, only 40 per cent of young people who were in state care at 16 had completed further education at ages 27–30, half the proportion in the population at large (Bryderup and Trentel, 2013). In the US, it is estimated that less than one in 10 care leavers obtain a degree (Okpych, 2012). There is limited evidence from Australia, but care leavers appear to be significantly underrepresented in tertiary education there too, particularly indigenous populations (Harvey et al., 2016). A number of issues are relevant to this issue, including young people's aspirations and qualifications, the expectations of adults and access to resources.

It is not clear how the aspirations of young people in care compare with those of their peers: a review of English and Welsh literature (Mannay et al., 2015) concludes that as a cohort, they have the same aspirations as others, but the 32 young people in the English YiPPEE case study (Cameron et al., 2011) demonstrated somewhat modest and general aspirations. US research (Stone, 2007), endorsed by that of Honey et al. (2011) in the UK and Flynn and Tessier (2011) in Ontario, Canada, suggests that young people in care have relatively high aspirations, but are often unable to achieve their goals, in line with Atkins' (2010) small-scale study of English working-class students taking essential or functional skills qualifications. It is imperative that attention be paid to opportunities for young people to enhance their academic qualifications beyond GCSEs in England: research suggests that with appropriate support, young people may be able to make up considerable ground in the final years of compulsory education from 16–18 (Driscoll, 2011), but many care leavers are forced to follow atypical and often prolonged paths in order to do so (Cameron et al., 2011; Driscoll, 2011; Harvey et al., 2016 in Australia).

Constrained financial circumstances (Allen, 2003; Wade and Dixon, 2006; Driscoll, 2013a), reduced support, greater social demands and increased independence in college compared with school (Driscoll, 2013b) lead to some English care leavers dropping out of further education. Care leavers in the US are much more likely to leave school with only a GED (General Educational Diploma) rather than a high school diploma, reducing their opportunities to progress to university (Pecora, 2012). US students from care backgrounds also remain more likely to drop out of higher education programmes than peers from similar socioeconomic backgrounds (Day et al., 2011). Despite higher levels of academic and social motivation and greater expressed willingness to access academic and personal support than their peers, US care leavers are likely to have reduced family support and enter higher education with poorer school qualifications than their peers (Unrau et al., 2012).

Factors influential in improving post-compulsory participation and attainment in addition to those discussed above include individually-tailored learning, strengths-based assessment and educational support, identification and treatment of mental health issues, financial support to engage in further or higher education and being in care longer (Ajayi and Quigley, 2006; Höjer et al., 2008; Stein, 2008; Pecora, 2012; Ferguson and Wolkow, 2012). The *By Degrees* study also found that the support and encouragement of birth parents was a significant factor associated with university entry (Jackson et al., 2005), but it should be noted that a significant proportion of the 129 care leavers entering university in that study were former UASC, who were more likely to come from home backgrounds in which parents had university degrees and education was highly valued, in contrast to the experiences of their UK-born peers (Ajayi and Quigley, 2006). In some other studies, the influence of birth parents has been found to be potentially negative, including where parents appear to lack interest in or understanding of young people's educational aspirations; where the family remains dysfunctional; or where young people regard their birth family as predominantly a source of stress (Geenen and Powers, 2007; Driscoll, 2013a).

Barriers to improving participation in further and higher education include the separation of education and care in professional disciplines, adults' assumptions that vocational rather than academic routes are more appropriate for this group of children and the tendency for immediate self-sufficiency to be given priority over young people's educational aspirations by professionals (Jackson and Cameron, 2012; Monserrat et al., 2013). The YiPPEE research identified the need for carers and social workers to place much greater importance on educational progress, for schools to demonstrate a more understanding response to the effects of young people's experiences on their engagement in school and for the use of multi-professional teams, including well-qualified teachers and career advisors to support young people's educational transitions. As discussed further in Chapter 7, for English care leavers, educational transitions at 16-18 coincide with disruption in other areas of their lives, including transition to the leaving care team and unsettled accommodation: preoccupation with planning for leaving care is likely to aggravate the stress of preparing for examinations (Fletcher-Campbell, 2008; Driscoll, 2013b). For Swedish young people, concern about accruing debt for living costs was the most cited structural barrier to continuing in education (Johansson and Höjer, 2012).

Johansson and Höjer (2012) use the concept of cultural capital to explain the barriers to care leavers' progression to further and higher education, as exhibited in poor ties to birth families, placement and educational instability, education pathways being ruled out by carers and poor support for educational trajectories at transitions. Likewise, Finnie points out the importance of drawing on the wider educational research literature, which demonstrates that cost is usually not a deciding factor in young people engaging in post-secondary education, provided that they are encouraged to value further education, are appropriately prepared for it and wish to continue their studies. His research with Canadian young people demonstrates that parental education is a much more influential factor than family income in predicting post-secondary education engagement and suggests that the decision to progress to higher education is generally made surprisingly early, highlighting the need for enculturation initiatives to promote genuine equality of access to educational opportunities (Finnie, 2012).

Outcomes for care leavers

Focus on extending young people's engagement in further and higher education is crucial for care leavers because poor educational qualifications render them particularly vulnerable to unemployment, exacerbating the high risk of social exclusion in adulthood faced by this group (Stein, 2006a; Jackson, 2007). Unemployment has disproportionately affected young adults compared to older workers in the most recent global downturn in the UK, (Wales, 2014), in line with developed economies in general (OECD, 2015). The proportion of 19-year-old care leavers not in education, training or employment (NEET) in England stood at 38 per cent in 2015 (DfE/NS, 2016b). It is difficult to compare these figures directly with the general population, because the statistics cover different age categories, but population statistics for 2015 show a NEET rate of 11.4 per cent for 18 year olds (DfE, 2016), although two points should be noted: first, that nine per cent of 19-year-old care leavers were NEET by reason of illness or disability and a further six per cent due to pregnancy or parenthood; and second, that these figures hide broader issues of underemployment, both in terms of working hours and the nature of young people's jobs (Gardiner, 2014). In Wales, the unemployment rate for care leavers is higher than in England or Northern Ireland, at nearly four times that in the general population (Mannay et al., 2015).

A similar picture emerges from US research. In Okpych and Courtney's comparison of over 500 young people from the Midwest Study with data from the Bureau of Labor Statistics' nationally representative sample of youth employment (NSLY97) (Okpych and Courtney, 2014), less than half of the care leavers were employed in their mid-20s compared with 70 per cent of their peers, and the average earnings of care leavers were approximately half that of young people in the general population, even after excluding young people who were not earning at all. There was no statistically significant difference in employment or earnings outcomes for care leavers with only a GED certificate compared with those with no qualifications. The study also found that care leavers earned less than their peers even when their educational qualifications were comparable, but higher levels of educational attainment were rewarded for care leavers by greater increases in average earnings, meaning that higher educational attainment is of greater benefit for care leavers than for their peers. Attaining a degree was particularly associated with significantly higher rates of employment and pay.

This is significant, because care leavers in English-speaking nations still 'generally experience deplorable life outcomes' (Lonne et al., 2009: 173), while the authors of the European YiPPEE study concluded from the data available that care leavers 'are over-represented in virtually every indicator of disadvantage' (Jackson and Cameron, 2010: 11). A Swedish study of all children born between 1972 and 1981 found that risks for attempted suicide, substance misuse, serious criminal offending and social welfare dependency at the age of 25 were six to 11 times higher than amongst the general population (Berlin et al., 2011). In Sweden, where many young people are placed in care in adolescence and for behavioural difficulties (particularly criminal delinquency) rather than on the basis of established familial maltreatment, those placed for behavioural difficulties are at particularly high risk of early death, criminal offending, mental health inpatient treatment and teenage pregnancy, as well as poor educational qualifications (Vinnerljung and Sallnäs, 2008). Girls, and young people who were older at placement, tended to have better outcomes in Vinnerljung and Sallnäs's study, the last point probably reflecting the fact that children exhibiting antisocial behaviour at an early age are at higher risk for poor outcomes in adulthood than children with later onset behavioural difficulties. Okpych and Courtney (2014) suggest that reasons for the marked disparity in earnings between US care leavers and their peers may include mental health problems, accommodation instability, early parenthood, residing in poor neighbourhoods with limited employment opportunities and low levels of human, social and economic capital. Data from the Midwest study found African-American care leavers experienced lower employment rates than their White peers. Higher levels of unemployment were also associated with young people who were not in foster care before transitioning to independence, while lower wages were associated with placement instability prior to leaving care (Hook and Courtney, 2011).

One-fifth of young people at the English homelessness charity Centrepoint[3] in 2010 were care leavers (Centrepoint, 2010), and a quarter of the 261 single homeless people surveyed by Crisis[4] in 2011 had been in local authority care (Reeve and Batty, 2011). In a study in three US cities, over a third of the 600 young homeless participants had been in foster care (Bender et al., 2015). Care leavers in the US are at increased risk of homelessness both through running away from care and through a dearth of independent living services (Fernandes-Alcantara, 2013; Davison and Burris, 2014), but the response has been hampered by inadequate data on homeless youth (United States Interagency Council on Homelessness (USICH), 2013). Bender et al. (2015) found homeless care leavers to have similar backgrounds to their homeless peers who had not been in care, but care leavers reported greater exposure to maltreatment and were homeless for longer, especially if they had a history of physical neglect. Their sample of 221 homeless care leavers suffered high rates of mental health needs, with 69 per cent meeting the diagnostic criteria for substance use disorder, 36 per cent for depression and almost 26 per cent for PTSD. An Israeli study of young people interviewed a year after they left had care at age 18 found that 24 per cent were experiencing housing instability and eight per cent had nowhere to stay (Sulimani-Aidan, 2015).

Care leavers also have a greater likelihood of involvement in the criminal justice system. 37 per cent of the young people aged 12–18 in custodial institutions in England and Wales in 2015–16 had a care background (Simmonds, 2016). Ministry of Justice research estimates that almost a quarter of adult prisoners were in care at some time in childhood; adult prisoners with a care background are also likely to have been arrested for the first time at a younger age and are more likely to be reconvicted after their release (Williams et al., 2012). Children in care in the US become involved in the juvenile justice system at rates of between seven and 24 per cent (Cutuli et al., 2016), with the risk increasing with age of entry into care, and higher for African-American children, boys, children with multiple placement histories and those in residential or group care. Similarly, maltreated Australian children are particularly likely to be convicted of an offence if they are male, Aboriginal or Torres Straight Islanders, experienced physical or emotional abuse, were maltreated from childhood and into adolescence and experienced out-of-home care (Malvaso et al., 2017). In a Swedish study, 37 per cent of male alumni from long-term care had received a sentence of imprisonment, forensic psychiatric care or probation after turning 20, compared with five per cent of the general population (Berlin et al., 2011). Reasons for the high proportion of care leavers in the prison system are many and complex, including attachment patterns, special educational needs and the prevalence of mental health difficulties, as well as an apparent tendency for structural criminalisation, particularly of those in residential care in the US and UK through early contact with police when staff struggle to manage young people's behaviour (see Staines, 2016).

Some specific associations between maltreatment and poor emotion regulation have been observed by researchers. In their study of over 360 undergraduates in the US, for example, Oshri et al. (2015) found that child victims of emotional abuse were more likely than their peers to exhibit impulsive behaviour (including alcohol or drug misuse, anti-social behaviour and failure to use condoms) and to experience difficulty in pursuing goal-directed behaviour when influenced by negative emotions. The likelihood of young adult care leavers exhibiting risky sexual behaviour and drug and alcohol misuse increases with greater placement instability, even after controlling for adverse childhood experiences (Stott, 2012). A systematic review of the literature on substance misuse provides a somewhat confusing picture in which young people in care do not self-report higher levels of marijuana or alcohol use than their peers but may be exposed to 'hard' drugs at an earlier age, and care leavers exhibit higher rates of diagnosis of drug and alcohol use disorders, with the transition from care possibly aggravating substance misuse problems (Braciszewski and Stout, 2012). A Swedish study drawing on national cohort data found rates of substance misuse for graduates of long-term care between four and seven times those in the general population, although this was reduced considerably when accounting for parental substance misuse (von Borczyskowski et al., 2013).

Maltreated children also appear to be at higher risk of re-victimisation in adulthood (Hocking et al., 2016). One theory to account for this is betrayal trauma theory, which arose from observations that memories of traumatic events are affected by the nature of the victim's relationship with the perpetrator. In general, victims of trauma will remove themselves from the perpetrator's reach, but where that is not possible, as in the case of children abused by their carer, victims may forget the trauma. However, victims of betrayal trauma in childhood are at higher risk of a range of negative physical and mental health problems, as well as of further betrayal trauma in adolescence and adulthood. Hocking et al.'s research suggests that an anxious attachment style partially accounts for this increased risk of re-victimisation, particularly that perpetrated by intimate partners on women, as such victims seek to preserve a close relationship rather than disengage. US research also confirms a significant association between a history of childhood sexual abuse (including rape) and engaging in transactional sex for adolescents with a care history (Ahrens et al., 2012) and it is estimated that around 70 per cent of sex workers in England have been in care (Centre for Social Justice, 2013). Rates of early motherhood among US care leavers are far higher than population averages (Stott, 2012). By the age of 25 or 26, almost 80 per cent of the female care leavers participating in the Midwest study had been pregnant, and nearly a third of female study participants had been pregnant by the age of 18. 72 per cent of young women and 53 per cent of young men in the study were parents at age 25 or 26, compared with 41 and 28 per cent of their peers in the general population respectively (Courtney et al., 2011).

There is limited literature on mental health outcomes for care leavers (Harris et al., 2010), but unsurprisingly given the mental health difficulties experienced by children in care, they are at much higher risk of mental ill health than the general population. A study of 708 White and African-Americans aged 20–49 from the Casey National Foster Care Alumni Study found that over 40 per cent of each group displayed symptoms of one or more mental health disorders, with no significant differences by ethnicity after controlling for demographic background, risk factors and experiences

in care (Harris et al., 2010). There is robust evidence of an association between child maltreatment and adult personality pathology, and US research
suggests some particular associations between types of maltreatment and
personality disorders, including between physical abuse and antisocial personality disorder traits; sexual abuse and paranoid, schizoid, borderline and
avoidant personality disorder traits; and emotional abuse and 'Cluster C'
traits (which include avoidant, dependent and obsessive-compulsive personality disorders) (Lobbestael et al., 2010; Cohen et al., 2014).

More worrying is evidence that many outcome measures are not currently improved through care. In a meta-analysis of studies from a range
of countries, Goemans et al. (2015) assessed the adaptive functioning, internalizing and externalising behavioural problems, and total problem behaviour of children in care. Although individual studies reported a variety
of outcomes, the larger studies (of over 80 children) showed worsening of
adaptive functioning during the periods studied, while longer stays in care
in this meta-analysis were not associated with improved outcomes. Similar
conclusions were reached by a systematic analysis of 31 papers from 11 cohort studies, nine of which were from the US and the remaining two from
Sweden and Portugal, comparing outcomes for children in out-of-home care
with maltreated children who were provided with in-home support services
(Maclean et al., 2016). There was no clear evidence of improved outcomes
through out-of-home care in 29 of 40 outcome measures, including academic achievement. Seven studies suggested worse outcomes for children
in out-of-home care, and only four evidenced benefits from removal from
home, although the authors warn of difficulties in interpreting the findings
arising from selection bias.

Assessment of the 'success' of care in improving outcomes for young people is extremely difficult given the absence of a control group, the differing
profiles of children in care in different nations and the likely correlation
between remaining in care for longer (rather than returning to family of
origin), severity of maltreatment and personal characteristics such as behavioural difficulties. A comparison of over 7,000 children entering foster care
in Denmark before the age of 13 took advantage of a change in policy in the
1990s allowing children to remain in care longer, and found that although
children spending longer in foster care had greater experience of hospital-
isation and poorer educational qualifications in early adulthood, they had
higher average pay and were less likely to be unemployed at 21 compared
with those who spent less time in care (Fallesen, 2013). In contrast, a Swedish
study of around 700 care leavers found very little evidence that a longer
time spent in care resulted in improved adult outcomes, save for a higher
likelihood of more than basic schooling by age 25 for young people in care
for more than two years (Vinnerljung and Sallnäs, 2008). Doyle Jr. (2013)
studied over 15,000 cases of children in Illinois who were borderline for
placement in care: his analysis suggests that placement in care increased the
risk of delinquency in adolescence for that group of children. Some recent

research in England and Wales suggests that care improves outcomes for most children (Hannon et al., 2010; Wade et al., 2010), although these studies are unable to draw on the large scale data available to US academics.

Conclusion

It is apparent that the challenges faced by children in care pervade every area of their lives and are often exacerbated by deficiencies in the care system. Emotional and behavioural difficulties, however, may not be readily ameliorated in care, given the developmental tasks of adolescence and the many disruptions to children's personal lives consequent upon entry into care. Educational attainment is a critical factor in the life outcomes of children in care, and it is probably also the factor that is most amenable to focused professional intervention. To the extent that outcomes for care leavers appear to have improved in England, it is likely that this is due at least in part to a concerted focus on children's educational attainment, coupled with greater support for children leaving care – including in relation to their education – introduced since the turn of the century. The following chapter considers what we know about how to improve the educational outcomes of care leavers both from existing literature and the CLET study.

Notes

1 Used to refer to education programmes primarily intended for 15/16–18/19 year-olds.
2 A behavioural screening tool based on self- and carer-report (Goodman, 2001).
3 A charity supporting homeless young people.
4 A national homelessness charity.

6 Closing the gap

Improving the educational outcomes of care leavers

Introduction

Despite the complexities of research in this area, evidence demonstrates that educational outcomes for children in care can be improved. Findings from the YiPPEE study suggest that the social democratic welfare scheme typical of Scandinavian studies promotes better educational outcomes for children in state care than the neoliberal regimes characteristic of the US and the UK, although the authors point out that both Sweden and Denmark appear to have moved away from the former towards the latter model in recent years (Johansson and Höjer, 2012). In the UK, there has been sustained attention by policy-makers to improving the educational attainment and wider life outcomes of care leavers since the turn of the century, and England is the only one of the five YiPPEE countries to have paid significant attention to the participation of care leavers in higher education through specific policy and legislation, providing care leavers with access to professional advice and financial support (Cameron et al., 2012). In England, research suggests that entry to care below the age of 12 generally has a positive impact in terms of children's educational attainment (McClung and Gayle, 2010), while in Scotland, there is evidence that outcomes are improving (Connelly and Furnivall, 2013), although the 'attainment gap' persists in both countries. In Wales, despite a variety of initiatives since devolution, noticeable progress has yet to be observed (Mannay et al., 2015). This chapter briefly reviews English and international initiatives to support the education of children in and leaving care before providing detailed discussion of the insights gained from the CLET study on supporting children in school and in their post-16 educational pathways.

Initiatives to support the education of children in and leaving care

Improving the educational outcomes of children in care in England became a policy focus through the New Labour (1997–2010) government's social inclusion agenda. Since 2004, local authorities' duty to safeguard and promote the welfare of children in their care has included promoting the child's educational achievement (Children Act 1989 s22(3A)). Children in care must be given the highest priority in arrangements for admission to maintained schools under the School Admissions Code, although of concern is that academies (institutions with greater autonomy from their local authority, a category making up an increasing proportion of schools) may be granted dispensation from this requirement by the Secretary of State for Education where there is 'demonstrable need' (DfE, 2014: paragraph 4). Local authorities may also require a maintained school, or request an academy, to admit a child in care even if the school is full, an important provision in enabling the local authority to meet its duty to ensure as far as possible that a child's care placement does not disrupt their education or training (Children Act 1989 s22C(7) and (8)(b)). 20 school days are allowed for allocation of a school placement in the case of an emergency. During the two years during which children are studying for GCSEs at age 16, their education should not be disrupted unless there is an emergency placement change: a placement change which would affect the child's education must be approved at a senior level in the authority (Care Planning, Placement and Case Review (England) Regulations 2010, reg. 10) and arrangements made to minimise disruption to the child's education (DfE, 2015).

Statutory guidance (DfE, 2014) stresses the importance of involving children in decisions and encouraging high expectations of children by social workers and carers. Head-teachers are advised that they should 'so far as possible' avoid excluding children in care, a more relaxed stance than in non-statutory guidance in force at the time of the CLET study describing the exclusion of children in care as an 'absolute last resort' (DCSF, 2008: paragraph 78). The effects of exclusion on these children can be catastrophic because of the interdependence of school and placement stability and the central role that school can play in promoting resilient adaptation and providing a 'normalising' environment (Martin and Jackson, 2002; Cameron, 2007). In 2014–15, children in care were more than twice as likely to be permanently excluded than all children (DfE/NS, 2017) and over five times as likely to face fixed-term exclusion.

Section 99 of the Children and Families Act 2014 (amending the Children Act 1989 s22) requires local authorities to appoint at least one person to promote the educational achievement of children in care, usually referred to as the 'virtual school head'. The school inspection agency Ofsted (2011) found the virtual school a potentially strong model to drive improvement, although some virtual schools did not support children beyond the age of 16 (Ofsted, 2012). Effective virtual schools supported schools in the best use of personal education plans, early intervention, managing attendance and educational engagement, and assisting individual children with specific difficulties such as negotiating the transition from primary to secondary school. They challenged schools to encourage high expectations of children in care and promoted schools' support for other professionals, including foster carers (Ofsted, 2011). Virtual schools appeared to be associated with increased attendance and reduced exclusion among children in care, increased understanding of educational matters among other professionals and ensuring that educational issues are central to care planning and review (Ofsted, 2012). Virtual heads considered, however, that there were still challenges in raising expectations of children in care in some schools and in supporting children placed outside the local authority area (Ofsted, 2012). The seniority and professional expertise of virtual heads was valued by schools, carers and professionals (Ofsted, 2012). It is as yet unclear what effect the increasing number of academies with greater independence from local authority control will have on the work of virtual schools or on the attainment of children in care attending academies.

A core aspect of the virtual head role comprises advising and supporting designated teachers, a statutory role with primary responsibility for promoting the educational attainment of children in care within schools (Children and Young Persons Act 2008 s20). The designated teacher has lead responsibility for helping school staff understand the factors affecting the learning of children in care, promoting 'a culture of high expectations and aspirations', ensuring young people are involved in setting learning targets and ensuring that carers appreciate the importance of supporting children's education (DCSF, 2009: 5). The designated teacher is also required to undertake a key role in enabling children to make a smooth transition to a new school or college and to manage engagement with relevant people and agencies outside the school, including carers, social workers and the local authority virtual school. The limited research on the role of designated teachers suggests that although some young people appreciated their support, a reluctance to be singled out could limit the extent to which young people would engage with them (Harker et al., 2004). Fletcher-Campbell (2008) concluded that the different facets of the designated teacher role may be best undertaken by more than one individual and that children in care need individually-tailored plans and a flexible approach to their negotiation of an education system that operates to established norms of progress.

Similar attempts to encourage joint working are evident elsewhere. In the US, the 2008 Fostering Connections to Success and Increasing Adoptions Act requires collaboration between children's social care and education services to improve the educational attainment of children in care, yet barriers to cross-agency working appear to remain (Zetlin et al., 2010; Noonan et al., 2012). Some states have implemented educational liaison programmes, through which case workers meet regularly with children to support their attainment; collaborate with teachers, social workers and carers; and monitor attainment and attendance, although there is limited evidence of their success (Weinberg et al., 2014). Ontario, Canada, has introduced a similar system of education professionals appointed by the child welfare agency to advise and support social care staff, and established a Child Welfare

Outcomes Expert Reference Group to improve outcomes for the educational attainment, resilience and successful adult transition of children in state care, within a wider policy drive to support vulnerable students (Ferguson and Wolkow, 2012).

There is a dearth of robust empirical studies supporting specific educational interventions in both the English and Scandinavian language literature (Forsman and Vinnerljung, 2012; Evans et al., 2016). Evans et al. (2016) conclude from a systematic review of English-language reports of studies using Randomised Control Trials that evidence of effective interventions is as yet inconclusive, although Forsman and Vinnerljung (2012) suggest that tutoring is the intervention most supported by the empirical evidence base. One-to-one tutoring by foster carers was found to improve some aspects of reading and maths skills in children aged six to 13 in comparison with a control group in a relatively small Canadian study (Flynn et al., 2012), while preliminary findings from a larger study, also from Canada, of a group tutoring programme delivered by university students demonstrated some success in word reading and spelling, but not mathematics or sentence comprehension, compared with a control group (Harper and Schmidt, 2012). Provision of one-to-one tuition in England was valued by children (Ofsted, 2012), but there is no longer dedicated funding to support it. Instead, children in care aged four to 15 attract the highest rate of Pupil Premium, money for targeted intervention to support disadvantaged groups, which is managed through the virtual school.

There have also been attempts in the UK to improve the accessibility of and support in further and higher education for care leavers. In addition to the legislative provisions set out in Chapter 2, which include financial support to the age of 25 to the extent required by care leavers' educational or training needs, care leavers in England are entitled to the 16–19 bursary and the Higher Education Bursary. A similar programme exists in the US under the Education and Training Voucher scheme, but support is variable from state to state and across institutions (Okpych, 2012). US research suggests that making foster placements available to 21 encourages engagement in higher education, but most young people will not be able to complete their degrees by that age, when most forms of support end (Okpych, 2012). Introduction of the charitable sector's Buttle UK Quality Mark for colleges and universities led to increased awareness of the needs of this group; however, the Quality Mark was discontinued after 2015, despite less than a quarter of further education colleges having achieved the award. A report on good practice in colleges awarded the Quality Mark stressed the importance of all staff having some understanding of the distinct needs of care leavers, regular review of policies with input from care leavers, networks through which to share good practice, a designated member of staff, targeted approaches to the engagement and support of care leavers, the availability of immediate support when needed and interagency collaboration with social care, health services and schools (NIACE, 2015). Recommendations in relation to good practice in universities also include designated staff, tailored interventions and financial support and input from care-experienced students, with additional stress on targeted outreach and widening participation activities and the importance of year-round accommodation (Rawson, 2016).

Supporting children in school: findings from the CLET study

'Success' as keeping children in school

Designated teachers identified advocating to keep children in school as a central aspect of their role, recognising the pastoral value of school at times of disruption in other areas of a young person's life by offering security, continuity and a sense of normalcy to young people whose lives may otherwise be unpredictable and unsettled (Dixon et al., 2006). Keeping a young person with very challenging behaviour at school helped to take pressure off a placement under strain. Some were sceptical as to the extent to which the introduction of the designated teacher role could reasonably be expected to boost educational outcomes, regarding its primary impact in terms of preventing exclusion:

> successful in we keep students in school, we don't exclude them...but whether they are actually making that progress...I think...the progress is better than it was, because they are in school (Ms Teal).
>
> that's what it's all about, keeping them here at school, making sure they are getting an education (Ms White).

For the most part, participants expected challenging behaviour from this cohort:

> *What have been the main issues...?*
> We have a lot of behavioural difficulties with some (Ms White).
> I think managing...their challenging behaviour. Maybe it's just been particular ones we've had (Ms Teal).
> it's mostly behaviour...if there are changes in placements or any disruption in that routine, I think we see the big difference in school...and probably the biggest part of my role is managing that in school, and trying to make the school experience as good as possible, and not really disrupted, if possible (Ms Rose).
> ...we've got a really good bunch, we've been very lucky, we haven't got any kids that are tremendously difficult to deal with (Mr Green).
> *Are there any particular priorities or challenges?*
> More on behavioural issues than anything else, if they don't like where they are placed they might cause some trouble (Ms Willow, Millbank College).

Designated teachers and virtual heads regarded advocating for young people as central to their role and both groups highlighted their work in ensuring appropriate school placement, monitoring attendance and preventing exclusions. The seniority of the designated teacher within the school was regarded as an important factor in enabling them to 'fight' (Mr Black) on behalf of young people to avoid permanent exclusion and/or access services to support their reinstatement in school. A number of participants mentioned instances of young people who would have been excluded from school had it not been for their care status and the designated teacher's persuasive influence on the head-teacher. Mr Brown thought 'you've got to also have some powerful influence...I think the designated teacher should be as senior as possible really', a sentiment echoed by Mr Brook:

> [s]ometimes you wonder, with some of the designated teachers, are they struggling to find their voice in schools?...but it's actually making sure really that designated teachers are appointed at that level of seniority, so they really have a voice, not just in supporting that particular child, but developing policy and strategy within the school.

Virtual heads also highlighted exclusion issues as central to their work and particularly the need to ensure that schools understand that permanent exclusions should not be imposed on young people in care. They, too, would step in on behalf of individual pupils to dissuade a head-teacher from excluding them. Mostly they felt they were successful but some felt that the environment was hardening:

> schools understand that exclusion is not an issue, it's not something that's acceptable for our looked-after children (Ms Ford).
>
> I think the main achievement for me and my team has been around attendance, in particular exclusions, we didn't have any permanent exclusions for like three years... (Ms Lea).
>
> We have a lot of our work characterised by crisis management, in terms of trying to support schools...either to keep children in school, or working with them to manage the move of a child somewhere else, rather than being excluded, and we are very good at that...it's getting more difficult...all our schools, basically, have gone academy secondaries... lots of things that are happening at the moment will probably lead to exclusions becoming worse (Ms Mason).
>
> ...we have too many looked-after children in the PRU, and they are sometimes our children who have been excluded outside the borough, and they come back to us (Mr Steel).

The fact that six of the young people in the study (Habib, Luis, Niall, Qadira, Riley and Unity) had been permanently excluded from school appears to support the view that not all schools are as sympathetic as they might be towards supporting children in care to stay in mainstream schools. So, too, does Ms Olive's observation that in some years the entire population of her special school for children with educational, behavioural and social needs was in care. For some young people, good quality alternative provision *could* be a lifeline: Ms Ford recounted her experience of a young woman who had suffered sexual abuse over some years:

> her behaviour at school became really, really, challenging, and she had lots of short term exclusions...she is now in a specialist residential school, and...she is just a different person...she is getting one-to-one tuition nearly all of the time.

A smaller, more relaxed and supportive environment with greater personal attention from staff can provide a chance to develop basic social and academic skills and gain confidence (see Poyser (2013) for a discussion of inclusion policy for children in care). That was briefly the case for Niall, who was beginning to flourish in a small independent school for excluded young people at the time of the initial interviews, but Habib was seriously let down by the alternative education provided for him after he was excluded for possession of drugs at school. He had some access to college but was only preparing for GCSEs in (he thought) maths and English. Although initially hesitant to criticise the provision when interviewed there in the first year of the study, he confided:

> I just want to study something that I'm going to be doing GCSEs in...I wish I was still in school....it's too laid back, they are too soft...some of my teachers don't even really come in...what time is it?...
> *It's gone twelve o'clock.*
> Yeah, some students are coming now, they are meant to come at nine o'clock...some teachers will wait for them. And it's hard on my education...it's taking the piss really.

Looking back in the final interview, Habib concluded '[t]hat place was shit'.

Once excluded from mainstream provision during a two-year GCSE programme (Years 10–11), it was not easy to return. Ms Coral explained

> if...they were meant to come to us for a twelve-week programme, by the time you've done that...to put them back into a new mainstream school, having missed most of the coursework, you are setting them up to fail. And schools won't take them towards the end of Year 10 or the beginning of Year 11, so they end up staying with us.

Ms Carmine also felt that out of sight was out of mind for many schools:

> normally what happens is once they are here they are here...I do have one or two schools that do come up and see me every week, and still

interested in their students, and then some just don't, I have to be prompting them to come and visit, come and look at the work, come and look at the progress.

'Success' as doing well

Luis was another participant who was dissatisfied with the limited curriculum and access to qualifications at his small school for young people with social, educational and behavioural difficulties, but he nonetheless persevered to gain adequate qualifications to enter college a year behind his peers. Habib progressed to college with his year group, but he was forced to study a subject he was not really interested in, and started again at level 1 (functional skills) in a new college with a new course the following year. Such determination was characteristic of many of the young people in the study. Those who were settled in school were proactive in seeking help to ensure that they had the best chance of attaining their goals:

> I have a French and Maths tutor…Because I was not failing, but I wasn't doing as well in French, and I just wanted to boost my Maths grade up…I asked the school and my social worker (Kayla).
> …my science teacher – I'm not really learning much from him, so I complained…Yeah, I said it out loud to my Head of Year so that she knows. And then [Miss Gold], she went and talked to my science teacher and then called my [foster] mum and hopefully it was sorted out (Jacinda).

Ms Ford, whose virtual school team attended all PEP meetings in schools to get to know the children personally, confirmed that 'certainly the older ones, are quite happy to ask for help, and accept help'.

In keeping with the depiction of UASC in the literature (Jackson et al., 2005; Jackson and Cameron, 2012), education was Bashir's highest priority. Having arrived unaccompanied from Afghanistan aged 12 or 13 with little prior education and minimal English, he was predicted the exceptional achievement of four A*s in his A levels (taken at age 18). He was extremely demanding both of himself and his school, demonstrating an insatiable appetite for study: 'I always think of myself "I have to know that", or if there's a topic I wasn't sure I go home research it all the time'. He was anxious for individual attention:

> The teachers are helpful, a lot, but…they have to give their support to everyone, which is not possible…that's why I want more support, one-to-one, because when I had it last year I could tackle any problems I had.

Despite receiving one-to-one tuition, Bashir was not wholly satisfied with his GCSE results:

> ...now I realise I could have done even better...I should have got all A*s...I could have done better in my English language...that's the only B I had...Say you get an A or something you can even do better again by getting a hundred percent, that's what I always wanted to do, be the best.

Adam too put all his energies into his schoolwork:

> it was Year 10 when I picked up, end of Year 10. And Year 11 I come back, I just thought "here I go, I'm going to take this" and everything, Eminem in my music, and I just done what I've got to do. Just worked hard...Now I'm happy, I think I'm one of the highest achievers the school's ever had in foster care.

A number of participants had curtailed their hobbies and social life to focus on their studies during the course of the research, including Tasmin, who said 'recently I haven't been doing anything because I've got a lot of home-work'. Often they felt that stigma still clung to them and/or that they had 'something to prove' to themselves or others. For Kayla and Adam, this related to breaking away from the cycle of failure they saw in their birth families. Kayla said 'I think I'm the only one in my family...who's gone this far in education...it's like I'm kind of making my own way instead of follow-ing other family traits instead'. Adam explained:

> I wanna go somewhere in life...looking at my...real family, I can see they ain't gone far in life, that's why they've got into these stupid situations. So basically I want to show other people that a boy who has basically lost four years of his education ...there's no reason why you cannot go far in life, and there's no reason why you cannot get good grades.

These sentiments resonate with those of others, such as the young people from the Swedish cohort of the YiPPEE study (Johansson and Höjer, 2012).

Raising expectations for the attainment of children in care

The CLET study provides evidence of a significant shift in professional attitudes in English practice when compared with earlier research findings that profes-sionals and carers did not prioritise education for children in care (SEU, 2003; Berridge, 2007). Ms Mason said that 'strategic priority number one is to raise attainment', and Mr Brook observed that 'the priority is always trying to raise achievement of young people'. In contrast, 'ten years ago...it was "can they be in school?"' (Ms Lea). Designated teachers were described as 'committed to try and get the best out of their children' (Mr Brook). Ms Olive stressed the importance of 'really high aspirations – "this is what you can achieve with your life"' for children who had always been told they were worthless. It appears that such attitudes are not, however, universal. Ofsted (2012) found that virtual heads felt that some schools were still not demonstrating high expectations for children in care, and, as reported above, children in alternative provision could effectively be 'written off'. Ms Carmine, for example, commented: 'I think they kind of used here as a holding space...rather than [Niall] becoming someone, and achieving, and being successful'.

Designated teachers in mainstream schools were at pains to point out that they saw the encouragement of high expectations not in terms of singling out children in care but rather as including them fully in a process of established good practice:

> it's part of my role for all our students...I know what these children should be capable of, and...we set ambitious targets above that...[for] all our students, so these students should be no different, and will be no different (Mr Black).
>
> it's something we do as a school, is high expectations of all of them... from everyone on SEN register to everyone in the school (Ms Rose).
>
> it's our duty to everybody, whatever their category. It's the same for our children in care, it's the same for our children who are on the special needs register, it's the same for our high flyers (Ms Gold).

However, evidence from the study suggests that while the desirability of high expectations for children in care has been absorbed by carers and social workers, not all have the necessary skills or understanding to support young people's education appropriately.

Young people generally felt that their carers were fully involved in their education:

> Sometimes I just tell her I've done it and I haven't...but...she knows because school tells her when I don't do homework...
> *Is that a good thing or a bad?*
> Yeah, because I wouldn't do it (Tasmin).

Often they were appreciative of foster carers who actively enforced discipline in their studying, and implementing strict rules when younger could translate into self-discipline as children matured:

> ...sometimes I get bored so I just...you know, leave it...usually when I go home, it's like you have to finish your homework before you do anything else, so I manage to do it (Kayla, first interview).
>
> I don't really do much outdoor activities at the moment, just because I have nine weeks left and I just want to finish my course...I don't really

go out in the weekdays, I go out on the weekends...don't have time to go out so much now (Kayla, third interview).

Where relationships with foster carers were strong, the family's work ethic could be highly influential on young people in the way that might be expected within birth families:

> *Do you have a particular role model in life...?*
> I would say my mum, foster mum...Because she works so hard...she's at uni, she's pushing herself to get better and stuff, and I think that's really good, and it's pushing me to do more as well (Jacinda).

Professionals, however, reported a more mixed picture in relation to the expertise and engagement of foster carers in educational matters. Although carers in Ironbridge were more involved in young people's education than they used to be, 'their own education is still very limited...We can get carers...much more readily...but having carers who are educated beyond a certain level is quite challenging' (Mr Steel). At Wadebridge

> We've got some very highly educated ones, but we've also got some for whom I would say that they have no personal experience of higher education...a lot of them find it very difficult to understand what levels of attainment are like, and what they should be expecting (Ms Ford).

Ms Olive described a 'strong ethos' of educational support in both foster and residential homes, but Ms Coral's observation that children placed in foster care were more likely to be supported in their education regrettably reflects the consistent findings of research (Berridge and Brodie, 1998; Jackson and Ajayi, 2007). Foster carers were not always readily engaged, however. Ms Carmine recounted of Niall's carer, 'I had to put my foot down and say "listen, you are his carer at the end of the day, you've got to be involved in what we are doing here"'.

Young people also reported that social workers placed high importance on their educational progress and for some the cumulative attention could feel overwhelming or maddening:

> *Is there anything you'd like to say about [being in care]?*
> There are loving people, and they try for your best...but...basically, social workers and key workers...all they've got is just education, education (Qadira).
> It's too much. Seriously. Every time my social worker sees me. Just about school, school...it's like "...that's important, that's your future"...I had enough in school, and when I come home the same stuff, it's every day (Sofia).

...she sits there telling me any level I get's not good enough, and it has to be an A*...I got a B in like English once, and I was like one mark off an A...and I was like "...you are a social worker...you didn't really do anything good with your life" and shut her up (Tasmin).

Most meetings all they think about is my education, and they want me to work and do things...I do get annoyed sometimes...because at my age I shouldn't be having meetings...to do with my life, so I do get stressed about it sometimes (Gilroy).

Young people's sense of pressure is understandable in the broader context of an education system heavily focused on measurement of progress, something virtual heads saw as central to their role:

it is about attainment and levels and what the schools are saying and the PEP targets and education targets and the emphasis is about attainment, and outcomes, quite frankly (Ms Lea).

Three times a year, we collect data on the educational levels of achievement of all our children, and so we are able to challenge if we think progress is not in place (Ms Ford).

We meet on a half-termly basis, we look at outcomes across the piece, and we discuss the progress (Mr Steel).

Virtual heads acknowledged that understanding educational processes was often challenging for social workers: 'I wasn't sure how much they understood of the possibilities post-sixteen...and also educational qualifications' (Mr Steel), reflecting Ofsted's findings (2012) that social workers' understanding of educational issues requires further attention. The virtual schools trained and supported social workers to 'hold schools to account much better' (Mr Steel) and in 'challenging the school, and making sure these are stretched and appropriate targets' (Ms Lea). However, young people did not always feel their social workers were able to give them educational advice:

Educational-wise I don't get any support from my social worker...She does talk about how my school is going and everything...but I don't get help in education...I don't think they know much because...she said I'm gonna be probably the second person that will be going to uni she knows (Bashir).
Do you think she understands about your education?
No. Not really.
Is she interested in education, do you think?
Don't know about that...but I don't think she knows what she's doing (Niall).

Overall, however, virtual heads felt that their efforts were paying off. Ms Lea said her virtual school had 'lots of kids at uni', and Ms Ford expected three of the 11 children in the penultimate year of school in Wadebridge to apply for university places. Support for this group was high on their agenda and Mr Steel described his intervention with one young man:

> I pulled him in here at the start of his A level courses, because I wanted to make sure he was doing appropriate courses, and I wanted to talk through his [GCSE] results…I wanted to gauge how hard he'd worked, and what the capacity was to improve.

Most of the young participants were actively considering going to university and spontaneously referred to their expectation of progression to higher education in interviews:

> *Do you think it's a good idea that young people should have to stay in education until they are 18…?*
> I think it's a good idea…like you'd waste your education if you don't go to college, because at the moment you are getting your education so you can get somewhere in future, so you can go to college, and on to university (Farouk).

Since children in care have preferential admissions status, some were in high-achieving schools where university entrance was the norm. Higher education has expanded significantly in recent years, so to an extent this may be a reflection of the expectations of their generation, or, in the case of UASC, of their family background:

> *What about your friends…Do you talk to them much about…future careers and things?*
> Yeah, me and my friend was talking about university the other day, like what were good ones, and talking about the one we visited. Yeah. Talking a lot about that (Tasmin).
> I want to be in school and have a good mark for stay at school…and go straight off to uni (Sofia, who had arrived in the UK eight months prior to the interview).

Sensitivity to young people's individual circumstances and aspirations

Sophia's comment illustrates that the reality for young people in care may not match the rhetoric of high aspirations and attainment. Data from the CLET study illuminate the tension in the literature between Berridge et al.'s suggestion that 'low achievement' is a more appropriate term than 'underachievement' for this cohort (Berridge et al., 2008) and the concerns of others such as Jackson that children's abilities have too often gone unrecognised or unfulfilled (Bentley, 2013; Jackson, 2013a). Ms Lea referred to measuring the attainment of children in care against an expectation that 'they have to be the same as everyone else': 'it's the Holy Grail isn't it, closing the gap'. While it is clear that the highest educational aspirations are appropriate for some of this very diverse group, such as Bashir (and see Bentley, 2013), for some other young people in the study, the promotion of 'high' expectations, where these were narrowly defined by access to university or entry to high-status professions, was more problematic.

In some cases young people appeared to be encouraged to aim for university entrance even though it did not seem to be an appropriate route for them, either because they were unlikely to achieve the necessary qualifications, or because university was not a helpful step on the way to achieving their career goals. Jacinda's foster carer, with whom she had an excellent relationship, had done her utmost to encourage her to take a traditional academic pathway, and Jacinda had done her best to comply – despite not knowing quite why university was a good idea. In the first interview she said 'I do want to go to university, but I don't know why I want to go on to university'. By the second, she had changed her mind, explaining 'I keep saying I don't want to go to uni, because I'm kind of scared in a way…if I can't cope with A levels then I definitely won't be able to cope with uni'. In the final year, Jacinda was much happier and more confident, having left school for college. She regretted the wasted year at school but still intended to go to university and held no grudge against her carer:

> she thought it would be good like, for a child in care to have done A levels, but when I changed my course she understood, and she was like well as long as I go to uni and do well.

Adam's school arranged for him to go to an Open Day at Cambridge University. He was thinking of studying Philosophy, Politics and Economics, although he had not achieved the government's benchmark grades at GCSE, and Mr Green acknowledged that he would have to be 'let down gently'. By the third year of the study, Adam had reverted to his original plans to go into construction. He had offers from three universities but felt no 'good' ones offered construction, and there was less work experience available in a degree course than through an apprenticeship. Unfortunately, apprenticeships were extremely competitive, and there were few opportunities still available because his focus on university entrance had delayed his consideration of alternative pathways. Gilroy confided a desire to attend university and study Sports Science only after the recorder had been switched off, which may have been indicative of his awareness that his ambition was unrealistic at that point, or perhaps it reflected a fear or previous experience of ridicule. At that stage of his life, Gilroy was living semi-independently after an incident in his foster placement, and he had dropped out of a level 2 (GCSE equivalent) Sports qualification at college, where his behaviour had been deliberately challenging. He was awaiting an appointment to join a local authority initiative with a local professional football team aimed at providing life skills and sport to care leavers at risk of becoming NEET (not in education, employment or training).

Michael offered the only apparent instance of a less academically ori-ented young person being steered gently in an appropriate direction. After his designated teacher, Ms Teal, had spoken to him about his career plans, he revised his goal. 'Originally I wanted to be a zoologist', he explained, 'but I changed my mind and want to be a zoo keeper, because I want to have more interaction with the animals'.

Professionals shared similar views as to the interdependence of students' ed-ucational attainment and pastoral well-being: in Mr Black's words: 'it is very, very difficult to compensate and deal with the emotional turmoil that these children are going through'. However, there were some differences of opinion as to the effect of promoting high-status aspirations among vulnerable cohorts through the somewhat aggressive mechanisms of target setting and monitor-ing. Some participants acknowledged that the focus on meeting targets might be a considerable source of stress for some young people: 'they should be meet-ing minimum target grades, all students should, and that's really hard, so the pressure is on those students' (Ms White). Both Ms White and Ms Teal held responsibility for students in care in Year 11 who had experienced a recent placement move or breakdown and were attuned to the likely effect that would have on GCSE performance. Ms Teal said of a student at Meadowpond:

> he's able and bright, and his predicted grades up until a couple of weeks ago were five A-Cs. He's got a good chance of getting five A-Cs, probably more than five, but with the placement breaking down I'm not sure now.

Similarly, a young woman at Clifton was not expected to get the GCSE grades she was capable of:

> We have one student who...is bright enough to be able to get a B... in some areas, but I suppose she's not very switched on...because of everything, I think, that's happened. She's moved foster placements quite a lot, this is her second secondary school, she started in Year 9, and her placement's just moved recently, and it's just really difficult, because the last priority, really, is her grades (Ms White).

While participants such as Adam and Jacinda readily accepted being steered into the most academic qualifications that they might realistically achieve, for others, there was a mismatch between their own ambitions and the expectations of professionals. In some cases, this difference served to highlight the extent to which young people's individual aspirations were communicated to or understood by designated teachers. Mr Black said of Devora: 'she's highly academic, we need to make sure, and she will, that she goes the usual path, A levels, university degree, off into the world of work'. However, Devora herself was clear that she wished to study Performing Arts at college, with a view to a career in drama, singing and dancing and that this had been a long-term ambition.

How and why the prevailing association of university entrance with success has arisen is unclear from this study and beyond its scope, although
it does reflect concern as to the precarious career pathways that are often the lot of young people with vocational qualifications as well a wider
privileging of formal academic qualifications over vocational skills in the
UK compared with other countries (Wolf, 2011; Baker, 2014), discussed
briefly in the preceding chapter. Possibilities include pressures on local
authorities to demonstrate improved levels of entry to higher education
by care leavers; traditional middle-class values held by teaching staff; assumptions as to the employment prospects for graduates; and the lack of
availability of good vocational training options (Wolf, 2011; Winch, 2012;
Foley, 2014). It is important, however, that professionals do not succumb
to the pressure of performance targets by failing to respect young people's
own interests and aspirations. Broader and more individual understandings of what constitutes 'success' may serve some young people better,
but it is also crucial that young people's attainment at 16 is not assumed
to represent their academic capabilities. The remainder of this chapter
considers the key issues which arose in relation to encouraging and supporting the young participants' educational attainment post-16: whether
school or further education colleges are best-suited to the needs of young
people, enabling a successful transition from school to college and the
support available at college.

Supporting young people's post-16 pathways

As Table 5.1 shows, most of the young participants' qualifications at 16 were
significantly lower than required to assure normative progression post-16
and entry into the labour market in adulthood. Transition at 16-plus was an
issue for all virtual schools in the study and virtual heads evidenced growing
attention to practice post-16, with Ms Mason commenting:

> I'm very concerned that we don't have adequate continuity and follow-
> through... detailed work around where they are going, are there issues...
> what can we do to support that educational establishment to keep that
> child, or maybe can we work with them to find something more appro-
> priate so they'll be more engaged...we've worked quite a lot to make
> sure the NEET figures improved, but there's still a lot of gaps from that
> transition from sixteen.

Virtual heads recognised that for policy reasons local authorities' focus has
tended in the past to be on GCSE attainment and the prevention of young
people becoming 'NEET'. At Wadebridge, Ms Ford described the 16-plus
transition as 'a bit hit and miss up to now', but 'targeted as an area for real
development', while Mr Brook referred to a need to refocus some of the
work, from 'supporting those young people post-16, who look as if they are

going to fall out of everything' to ensuring that able students fulfil their potential at A level and through entry to higher education.

Although at Stonycross there was concern that 'sixteen to eighteen is the stage where they can become very disaffected, lose track, and lose focus (Ms Mason)', there was also an emerging recognition that young people can often make up considerable ground post-16 and commitment to enabling them to do so. In The Valleys, Ms Lea commented that 'by Year 12, 13…more of them have picked up or come back into education, because that is the push'.

Resonating with the focal model of adolescence, Ms Lea explained:

> I know there's a lot more success when they get older because maybe they can manage what's happened better, but us expecting them to be brilliant at 16, like everybody else is, is quite difficult…it's not because they haven't got the ability, or they are not willing, it's about what's happening in the processes in their lives, and they are trying to manage all of that and do school.

Mr Brook thought:

> it is very important to try and give…young people…a second chance post-sixteen… young people who haven't really done very much at all… with support, by seventeen, eighteen, have managed to sort of find their feet and begin to gain some… qualifications.

School or college

The inherent difficulties for schools in reconciling the need to 'make allowances' and provide strong and consistent pastoral support for this cohort with the focus on academic attainment appeared to become most acute when considering entry to school 'sixth forms' or further education colleges when young people are 16. The professional participants generally considered that remaining in school had significant advantages for these children in terms of continuity of relationships, a sense of security and ongoing support. Ms Ford stated 'I would definitely prefer to have them in schools', and Ms Lea explained 'there's more established support in school'. Mr Brown stressed the enormity of the 16-plus transition:

> the last thing we want, and you've got to rein some teachers back from this…is them to leave. They are much better staying with us…Because we all know that transitions are awful, and that transition, from sixteen to seventeen is terrifying, and if they can stay with us they've got some sort of stability.

He thought that at college

> you'll just be anonymous, no-one will know you…they won't…particularly care about you, but in school we know you, you've got people who

have built a very strong relationship with you, and they will look out for you and make sure things go well.

Ms White said 'particularly if it's a vulnerable student we will do our best to keep them here if that's what they want', while Ms Gold reflected on Imogen:

> I think she'd be more successful here…There's something quite comfortable about the [Queen's] environment for the girls…I think she might get lost a little bit [at college]…she had talked about childcare…that's a vocational course that we offer here, so she could remain with us, which is where I think she feels safe…Because I think she is not so brave…

Ms White related concerns about Gilroy:

> he's not as confident, and he interprets things differently to other students, the maturity isn't quite there yet…So I would worry about him leaving… So we will get him to apply to the sixth form, probably as a back-up plan, anyway, so that he can come back and be in a safe environment.

There were two factors which might stand in the way of young people remaining in school, however. First, while some, such as Callum, were apprehensive about leaving school ('I know everybody here, I know all the teachers, and, you know, I didn't want to go to college where I knew nobody'), others were attracted by a new start and greater independence, or struggled to conform in school:

> maybe they've had enough of that school, and the experiences, and everybody just wants them out of the door, they've done their exams now, thank God…you need a fresh start, it would be better for you to go to college (Ms Lea).

Ms Teal described 'leaning on' her head-teacher to fund a college place for a care leaver:

> If she'd have stayed here she'd have been a permanent exclusion, because she was only fifteen going on eighteen. She really didn't fit in school anymore…She won student of the year at college.

Second, schools were often unable to offer suitable curricula. While there were admissions criteria for progressing to 'A' levels in the sixth form, all of the schools appeared to have some form of vocational courses on offer. However, these were relatively limited compared with the provision available at further education colleges and often did not provide the same range of practical experience. Woodhall probably offered the widest variety of vocational courses, but Mr Brown explained: 'We have really good vocational provision, but we just cannot do some of the specialised vocational stuff', and Mr Green said: '[w]e like them to stay...but we've got a woefully bad level 2 offer'.

Some schools were very creative in attempting to give their students the best of both worlds. Ms Gold, for example, had supplemented a childcare course in school for one young woman with additional input from a college, to fill up her timetable and because she was not handling school very well. Such compromises allowed young people more freedom and access to more suitable programmes of study, whilst still enabling them to keep the continuity, familiarity and support available at school. Similarly, Ms Teal could arrange for joint attendance at Meadowpond and the adjacent special school, which offered some level 1 opportunities. She explained:

> we are quite small, and we are quite able to make exceptions...if we thought that the placement was good, and the child couldn't make the transition easily, and he was going to be very upset and anxious about it, we'd do all we could to keep him here, and to find a curriculum in the sixth form for him or her.

A perverse consequence of children in care having preferential admissions status is that high-performing schools are likely to have fewer vocational opportunities post-16. A number of designated teachers expressed concern that it would not be fair to keep students in the sixth form if they were not sufficiently academically able or prepared: 'if they haven't coped with GCSE we don't want to put them into a course they are not going to survive' (Ms White); 'we love our girls to stay with us into the sixth form...it's important though that students don't take on an AS/A2 course without having the grounding, because actually that wouldn't be kind' (Ms Gold). Ms Ford concluded 'if they want to do vocational-based courses, which quite a few of them do, then we have to look at college provision'.

Where young people's grades were not good enough to remain at school or to access their preferred college courses, there was generally provision at those colleges to start at a lower level (National Vocational Qualifications start at level 1 while GCSEs are at level 2). Yet previous research (Driscoll, 2011) points to the potential drawbacks in terms of loss of motivation and purpose when young people who have underperformed are forced to continue at a lower level of qualification than is commensurate with their ability. There are no universal requirements for care leavers to be given priority in admissions arrangements at colleges, although this was something a virtual head had raised with Ms Maple at Millbank College, and arrangements for transition to and support in further education colleges appeared underdeveloped.

Transition to college

Notwithstanding references in the statutory guidance (DCSF, 2009) to the role of designated teachers in helping young people make a smooth transition to college, liaison between schools and further education (FE) colleges appeared surprisingly limited. For some schools, contact with FE colleges of any kind seemed to be quite a recent development. Accordingly, there was little or no concrete knowledge in schools of what support might be made available for students. Colleges were seen as to a certain extent in competition with school sixth forms, and there was perhaps a measure of mistrust of the FE estate. Colleges also varied as to the contacts they made available to schools, with one communicating through their marketing department rather than allowing ready access to tutors. Ms Coral thought 'it would be good to meet with the college...but that's never happened', while Mr Green had tried on numerous occasions to talk to the college Elliott had attended on his behalf but had received no response to his communications.

For the most part, designated teachers appeared to regard the role of liaison with colleges as within the remit of the social services leaving care team, and schools did little more than send the student's academic record and references on request. Ms Willow at Millbank College observed that the college worked well with social care but found it difficult to get information from feeder schools. Some schools undertook transition planning work with their care leavers: Meadowpond, for example, arranged for young people to visit or undertake sessions at the local college, but with the move to the leaving care team, the school would become less involved. This was likely to be particularly the case when the young person was looked after by a different local authority than that to which the school belonged, and the local authority were seeking further education provision closer to home.

These are areas in which there is significant potential for virtual schools to facilitate smooth transition arrangements for young people and where necessary advocate on their behalf, but virtual heads reported varied practice. Mr Brook, whose virtual school was extending beyond 18, considered that Riversmeet had good contacts with local colleges, but elsewhere the transition was more problematic. Ironbridge had very recently extended to 18, and Mr Steel had started to focus more on post-16 work, but in the Valleys and Stonycross post-16 education was the responsibility of a different team. Ms Mason commented that one of Stonycross' priorities was 'a better system for continuity between school age children and sixteen-plus', because 'when you look at what actually happens when they come out of the virtual school...then it kind of just gets lost'.

Virtual heads highlighted establishing links with colleges as a priority and had given the issue considerable attention. However, as care leavers' results improved, they were 'becoming more choosy' and 'shopping around' (Mr Steel), requiring the virtual school to establish new relationships with more institutions. Ironbridge also had a high proportion of older young people out-of-area and had appointed an advisory teacher based in the county in which most of those children were placed who facilitated their transition to colleges and worked with the post-16 social work team within the borough.

Designated teachers in non-mainstream settings – usually the head-teacher – were much more focused on transition planning than their colleagues in mainstream schools, but this was something they undertook for all their children. A number of participants from alternative providers would have liked to provide ongoing support to 18 for young people: Ms Tan thought: 'we should go on to eighteen, because our kids aren't old enough to go out into the big wide world, in so many ways'. In some respects, there is much that the mainstream sector could learn from such providers because they have long been used to dealing with resistance by colleges to taking on the young people from their institutions. As Mr Grey observed: 'they only want the straightforward ones at college, it's cheaper'. All non-mainstream participating designated teachers also focused on providing the social skills young people would need to cope in college and were adept at putting together packages that would allow a gradual transition to provide some continuity at the outset. The Grove, for example, kept some children on a part-time basis concurrently with the first year of college, to enable them to make a more gradual transition. Ms Olive and Mr Grey both stressed the importance of being proactive in seeking timely indications from local authorities as to whether a child would stay in the area after 16 or be returned to their home authority in order for concrete educational plans to be made.

Support at college

Although the introduction of the 16–19 bursary has prompted payment of greater attention to this group in FE colleges, the support available appears to be patchy and the mechanisms through which it is delivered varied. 'Drop-out' rates from college were reportedly high, for a number of reasons. Ms Ford observed:

> I think schools are very good at supporting, and I won't say bending the rules, but perhaps being a little bit more sympathetic, and colleges have hard and fast rules…they kept on saying "…this is college policy, if their attendance rate has dropped below 85 per cent they are out".

Mr Steel confirmed that

> when they go into FE colleges it's about…getting them to actually turn up in the morning on a regular basis…Because the ones that are staying on in school are much more likely to be the ones that are doing level 3 qualification and are more focused.

Of the 11 young people in the study who went straight to college after GCSEs, four (Elliott, Priya, Riley and Unity) dropped out while a further two (Gilroy and Niall) were excluded for their behaviour. Despite Ms Gold's concerns, Imogen had a good attendance record at college and was studying level 2 Childcare in the third year of the study, having successfully completed level 1; she was planning to remain until she attained level 4. Priya, Unity and Riley all had patchy or disrupted school attendance records. Unity simply said 'college ain't really my thing'. Priya did not know what she wanted to do for a career but had attended a beauty therapy course 'for a bit'. Riley appeared to have difficulty settling on a career path, switching from Public Services to Hair and Beauty, but starting the latter course too late to catch up with peers. In the final year of the study he had failed the army's Combat Medical Technician exams and was planning to return to college the following year if he did not pass on retaking them. Ms Teal was aware that at least two of the five or so care leavers from Meadowpond had dropped out of college. Neither had remained in Meadowpond's local authority area: both had been moved to independent living placements in their 'home' authority.

About a quarter of the Ironbridge students dropped out of college, an issue that was the responsibility of the post-16 social work team, who could request the assistance of the virtual school should they choose (Mr Steel). This proportion was very similar to that at Eastside College, where by March the 60 care leavers enrolled in September had been reduced to 45. In contrast, the retention rate for care leavers at Forest Hill College in the year of the interview was 95 per cent, higher than the overall college rate. This had been the result of focused attention to the issue, although Ms Oak pointed out that there were some circumstances, such as placement moves or personal circumstances militating against the engagement of a young person, that were beyond the control of the college or the virtual school. She concluded that 'it would be a lot harder...if we didn't have good relationships with the virtual schools', but 'it isn't difficult...once you start having the conversations'.

Often there was no equivalent of a designated teacher in colleges. One of the colleges in Ironside had a named member of staff for care leavers, but only the smallest of the three colleges in Wadebridge had a safeguarding officer. Ms Ford had 'a very close relationship' with her, and she would provide a point of contact with individual heads of departments and facilitate meetings. In the other two colleges, it was a case of 'having to build a relationship with the individual course tutors' (Ms Ford).

Colleges, for their part, found communication with local authorities challenging, with Ms Oak saying

> I struggle sometimes with...knowing who to speak to, and knowing... what's available for our looked-after children from the virtual school, and what support's in place for them...

Although observing that it would be helpful to have more information about young people and communication channels within local authorities, Ms Oak took the view that the responsibility lay primarily with colleges:

> at the end of the day the people that have to take responsibility is the college; they are our students and...for the time they are with us they are our responsibility, so we do need to be the ones to take that role...

because we are, I suppose, in many cases, the...closest thing to a support network that that young person will have.

Not all colleges appeared to take a similar stance, however. One of the colleges at Wadebridge was so big that 'they don't even know the students on some courses' (Ms Ford), while at another:

> [the tutor] had no empathy whatsoever, no understanding whatsoever. He just said – "well, he's an adult now...I tell him what you've got to do, if he chooses not to do it that's his problem"...despite having had a meeting to try and explain the kind of extra support that was needed, it was obvious that this chap was never going to be in a position to provide it.

Ms Tan pointed out that this attitude was very different from that at school for her EBD students, where a lot of work was undertaken to engage students:

> a lot of our children end up as NEETs, because they get lost after that... we need to say..."you come in here and discover what you need in your college to make these children's lives work better".

Ms Oak observed that it would be constructive for Forest Hill College to be informed of crisis points in a young person's life, providing the example of a young woman with emotional and behavioural difficulties who was facing disciplinary proceedings in college, but the college had not been informed that the local authority had started the process of her leaving her carers: 'I think if we had known before...it would have helped us to help her'.
    Ms Willow at Eastside College had a similar experience:

> one boy...he refused to keep coming, and we found out that he had history that hadn't been shared with us until we'd actually decided he wasn't staying...we hadn't linked up to the borough...So we did give him another chance...He did one whole year...got into more problems, and then he left.

Among the three colleges represented in the study, there was considerable variation in the degree of development of services specifically for care leavers. Prior to the introduction of the 16–19 bursary for care leavers, it appears that some colleges relied on professionals to inform them of students' status and care leavers were often identified only once a problem emerged. Eastside College had a single designated opportunities coach for care leavers, Ms Maple; at Millbank College, there was a team of 10 in safeguarding, of which Ms Willow, the learner services manager, was responsible for care leavers. The most developed support framework was at Forest Hill College, where the director of learning services, Ms Oak, took responsibility for care leavers, reflecting a similar level of seniority to that required for a designated teacher in schools. The total population of Forest Hill was just under 12 thousand students, of which about 4,500 were aged 16 to 18, and 45 of those (one per cent) were care leavers. Ms Oak commented on the complexity introduced by the number of different local authorities with which she dealt, but she had initiated partnership agreements with local authorities. Where these were in place, either advisory teachers from the virtual school or social workers were based in the college for the first six weeks of the academic year to support young people's transition into college.

Support for care leavers started at interview because in Ms Oak's experience 'by supporting the transition to college we are far more likely to retain them'. Retention strategies included early introduction of the young person to a member of the college student support staff by the local authority case worker, so that there was an immediate and familiar point of contact within the college; enabling young people to make appointments with, and meet, their social worker at college; inviting local authority staff to any disciplinary or other meetings; and weekly reporting of attendance to virtual heads. Forest Hill also combined the course reviews young people undertook with their tutors with PEP reviews with their social worker so that they did not have to endure two similar meetings.

A scheme that Ms Oak regarded as particularly effective and employed with a number of vulnerable groups was an enhanced induction process, in which care leavers as a group were given a talk from the student support team about what support the college offered and ensured that they all completed their bursary application forms. The college highlighted to young people the practical support available, such as supporting the virtual school where a placement move was anticipated, when the college could, for example, press for reconsideration based on travel difficulties, or if necessary use learner support funds to finance their fare. What emerged from Ms Oak's account was a strong sense of the importance of attention to the everyday details of a young person's life and a willingness to advise and advocate for that young person in the same way that designated teachers described. The example of Forest Hill College demonstrates that there is considerable potential for the further education estate to facilitate good transitions for young people from school to higher education or employment where colleges are willing and able to work with local authorities and to take time to understand the individual challenges faced by young people.

Conclusion

For the most part, young people expressed a strong appreciation of the educational opportunities that care had opened up for them. Habib commented 'I wouldn't have got nothing, hardly ever went to school'; Adam said his prospects 'are much better, a hundred percent, I'm going to school more, I've got a place to study', and he also explained 'if you want to work hard and you know nothing bad's going to happen or whatever then you can work hard'. Kayla thought: 'if I wasn't in care then I don't think I would be motivated to anything, I wouldn't have a mindset of what I wanted to do'. These comments are in line with other evidence of young people considering that care enhanced their educational prospects compared with remaining at home (Sladović-Franz and Branica, 2013; Sebba et al., 2015).

Internationally, the low educational attainment of children in care and often high proportions of children entering care in adolescence renders attention to flexibility of provision and continuing high aspirations post-16 of particular importance. The evidence of the CLET study suggests that young people over 16 in England are currently better supported at school than in college in most instances, although it is important to bear in mind that the more academically successful young people are more likely to remain in school. Internationally, similar considerations will apply in relation to balancing the advantages of young people remaining in a familiar and supportive school environment versus those of a fresh start and greater independence, and similar challenges in avoiding locking young people into vocational or non-academic pathways before their academic potential is fully apparent.

As their results improve, English care leavers are able to access a wider range of educational institutions, but enabling them to do so will require considerable knowledge and expertise on the part of their corporate parent. Some FE colleges appeared to be at an early stage in communicating with local authorities to provide appropriate support for care leavers. Social care authorities internationally need to ensure they have robust links with education services and continued specialist educational support for young people to 18 and beyond. Although larger institutions may face greater difficulties in attending to the individual needs of young people, there is also greater scope for the development of significant expertise and specialist services and for close collaboration between such institutions and social care services. This is, however, an area in which research is lacking.

The model of the virtual school appears to be a successful one in its ability to promote collaboration between education and social care and provide continuity of support to young people throughout their educational career, regardless of changes of education and care placement and geographical moves across local government boundaries. However, while there is some encouraging evidence of higher achievement among some groups of care leavers, it is crucial that in promoting the attainment of successful young people, the needs of those who are most at risk of social exclusion in adulthood are not forgotten. The following chapter considers the great variation in young people's educational trajectories in the context of multiple transitions concurrently in all area of their lives.

7　From care to independence

Negotiating multiple transitions

Introduction

The data gathered from both young people and professionals in the course of this study attests eloquently to the complexities in all domains of the lives of young people ageing out of care and to the interdependence of their experiences in education and in care. I have situated these experiences within the developmental context of adolescence because this is a time during which all children undertake core developmental tasks as well as undergo key life transitions. The focal model of adolescence (see Chapter 2) posits that adolescents attend to the developmental tasks of adolescence consecutively and may struggle to cope with multiple concurrent challenges (Coleman, 2011). The focal model helps to explain the impact of late entry into care, placement instability, concurrent transitions in varying areas of young people's lives and the renegotiation of birth family relationships on reaching adulthood on young people's educational experiences and outcomes. Strengths of the model include that it can be applied to the experiences of all young people without singling out those with specific deficits or vulnerabilities, it acknowledges the universal developmental tasks of adolescence and it respects the agency of young people in constructing their own adolescence and managing the issues they confront.

In this chapter I first summarise young people's educational trajectories over the three years of the study before considering their multiple experiences of transitions in all areas of their lives. I draw on attachment theory and on the focal model of adolescence to help explain why this particular group of young people is especially likely to need additional time and support during adolescence as they grapple with multiple challenges during a key developmental stage. I discuss the primacy of relationships in adolescence and the effect of young people's reevaluation of their relationships with their birth and foster families on their decisions, actions and attainment in the years leading to legal majority. Next I assess young people's resilient adaptation based on the evidence of the study using Stein's categorisation of care leavers, with particular reference to their sense of self-reliance, and I use this as a means by which to explore their divergent trajectories. Third, I discuss young people's progression to independent living, their choices and anxieties around this stage of their lives. In conclusion, I briefly assess their future prospects in the context of those of their peers in an age of 'emerging adulthood'.

The polarized trajectories of young people

As the study progressed, the future appeared more daunting to young people and their prospects more uncertain. For some, this was the consequence of the near-inevitable setbacks associated with competitive career choices, such as becoming a doctor (Bashir), actor (Devora) or footballer (three of the young men). These issues may apply to many of their peers too, in the context of an identified misalignment of young people's career aspirations with opportunities in the labour market (Mann et al., 2013). However, most of the young people in this study were disappointed that in their own estimation they had not achieved qualifications in line with their academic potential. Moreover, they were juggling multiple transitions in their lives over the two to three years that I followed them, with simultaneous transitions in care, from the looked-after children team to the leaving care team and for some, to the transitions team (for young people requiring additional support after the age of 18); in accommodation, with moves from foster or residential care to semi- and/or fully independent living; in education; and in their personal lives, with leaving care providing them with an opportunity to reestablish relationships with their birth family – for better or worse.

Young people's prospects were highly divergent. By the end of the study (when they were 18), one-third (seven) of the group were not in employment, education or training (NEET), in line with national statistics for care leavers at age 19 at that time (DfE/NS, 2013). Bashir could confidently be expected to attain the grades he needed to attend university (although he had not obtained an offer to study Medicine, as he had hoped), Kayla would probably go to university, and Adam might also do so. Tasmin was not interviewed at age 18 but appeared to be on track to attend higher education should she wish to do so, and potentially Sofia might also do so if she successfully completed college. Imogen and Jacinda both planned to attend university but would take another year or two to acquire the necessary qualifications.

Table 7.1 shows the developing aspirations and plans of the young people over the course of the study in so far as they could be gleaned from interviews, given that only 10 young people participated in the final year of the study.

Transitions in multiple domains of young people's lives

The CLET study focused on a period of transition in education for all young people in England, but for care leavers this is likely to coincide with changes in their personal life. Mr Brook described 'a triple whammy, in terms of disruption', referring to young people leaving school, moving from

Table 7.1 Young people's changing plans over time

Name	Plans year 1	Plans year 2	Plans year 3	Comments
Adam	Building/public services	PPE at Oxbridge? Then business	University/ apprenticeship, construction	'I don't care if I hate what I do... I want the qualifications and the money. Then... caring for other people... That's what I want to do, charity work and stuff'.
Bashir	Medicine	Medicine	Medicine: offer Biomedical Sciences	'I didn't know it was going to be that hard to get into university'
Callum	Considering plumber	Considering plumber	Carpenter? Construction boring	Wants to stay at school another year to do new cookery course. 'I don't know what to do to be honest, but a chef, I suppose it could be good'.
Devora	Singer/actress/ dancer	Performing arts BTEC	Three rejections for drama/musical theatre, awaiting fourth	'It's all I've wanted to do...Since I can remember'. 'Plan B is to take a year out... travelling, volunteering ...And just get work ...because I need to support myself'.
Elliott	Footballer/fire service	Dropped out of college	NEET, plans unknown	Excluded from sports college (immigration).
Farouk	Footballer/ accountant	Footballer/media	Unknown but back in college	
Gilroy	Coaching; 'too old' for footballer	Sports Science at university	NEET, plans unknown	Year 2: 'I don't know what I'm going to do yet' – not thinking past '18' project.
Habib	Electronics	Carpentry level 1	Royal Marines, meanwhile Hospitality and Catering level 1	'I felt pressured...they [carers] were like "if you change this course what are you gonna do next week?"...And I had too much pride...I told them like I will finish this course...I can't do a three year course, I'd just lose interest'.

(Continued)

Name	Plans year 1	Plans year 2	Plans year 3	Comments
Imogen	Child care (nursery)	Psychology at university	Nursery teacher	Year 2: 'later on, I want to be a child psychologist…My sister does psychology in uni'.
Jacinda	Children's therapist/ art teacher/ photographer	'I've been babysitting …it's not as…I thought…, working with children'	General Health and Social Care BTEC; planning to go on to university to study Nursing	Year 1: 'help out people that were fostered, because I understand them …but I don't think I would get to it, because I'd have to pick psychology'; 'I had a therapist myself, and I really liked her, and then she really inspired me.' Foster mother suggested child nursing.
Kayla	Performing arts/sports psychologist/ sports therapist	Coaching or sports psychology	Sports psychologist/ drama therapist	'I want to work with people who are in difficult situations, like I was'; 'If I do a Masters I want to do drama therapy… so I can understand'.
Luis	Actor/plasterer	Media at college		Drama/music: 'I don't think I'll be so successful at them things…because I wouldn't have much experience…like camera crew, I'd be more successful…'.
Michael	Zoo keeper			Year 1: 'Originally I wanted to be a zoologist, but I changed my mind [after designated teacher input] and want to be a zoo keeper, because I want to have more interaction with the animals'.
Niall	Apprenticeship in plumbing	College/NEET	NEET, plans unknown	'I've got to go to college so I can get a level two in my reading and writing' (Year 1).
Ollie	College-cooking; to go to library by himself		NEET (disability)	Will be dependent all his life. 'I want to go college, I don't want to come here no more…'cos it's for children…I want to help some people…I like working with children'

Priya		Beauty therapy 'for a bit'	NEET	'Of course I want a career. I just don't know what I want to do'.
Qadira	Considering running her own beauty business in the long term. Looking for job/ apprenticeship in meantime	Training in a hairdressing salon/ applying for jobs, retail, everything	NEET Looking for jobs: 'Any jobs, retail, anything'	Year 3: 'I've gone sort of off beauty and hairdressing… I'm trying to get myself on track to go college and get a job or something, you know? I never thought I would get to this point, but I have, so it's good'. Would still like to run her own business but hasn't thought further about that: 'No, still young, still got time'.
Riley	No interview year 1	Public Services level 2 BTEC for fire or ambulance service	NEET Combat medical technician, job for couple of months	Has to retake army exam: "if they don't accept me then I will go back to hair and beauty' [level 2]. Job hunting: 'I did have one, as bar staff, but I got made redundant. It got shut down'.
Sofia	Fashion designer 'I don't have any other plan'			'It's very strange because I remember the first day when I come to school…I forget everything when I do textiles, and everything just go and you focus on what I'm doing.
Tasmin	Psychology: (carer's son did A level); previously teacher / midwife/ work with children	Considering accountancy: 'I really like doing business [studies]'		[SW] 'said that like being a midwife wasn't a good job, she kind of put me off'. 'I got onto a course to do health and social care…it was like everyone that failed their GCSEs horribly… so I was like "I don't want to do it, I want to achieve better than that"'.
Unity	NEET applying for admin apprenticeships			I was doing a childcare course…but I didn't complete it…obviously I'm just going to keep my options open, I don't know yet; sewing/soft furnishing 2 hrs/week.

foster care to semi-independent or independent accommodation and losing their social worker in moving to the leaving care team. Although specialist leaving care services have been associated with increased entry into further education and higher numbers of care leavers in employment or training (Hai and Williams, 2004; Dixon et al., 2006), a number of professional participants expressed concern that preparation for GCSE qualifications often coincided with planning for leaving care and moving to college, exacerbating the considerable stress young people were already under. Mr Brown spoke of young people feeling as if they had been 'dropped' when they transferred to the leaving care team. Ms Olive had experienced increasingly in the recent past that arrangements for young people who had been assured of continuity ('yes, you'll stay in this foster care until eighteen, yes...you can attend a local college where you are living now') might change with the change of staff, sometimes triggering behavioural problems. Some participants also expressed concern that post-16 teams were not fully staffed by qualified social workers and that the knowledge and education of some staff 'is sometimes quite limited' (Mr Steel). Wadebridge and another local authority had disbanded their leaving care team in favour of social work continuity; professionals who had experienced these arrangements felt that they worked better.

Designated teachers and virtual school staff recognised that sometimes it was unrealistic to expect young people to perform to their maximum academic potential in the face of placement uncertainty and disruption, when their grades were likely to be their 'last priority' (Ms White). Ms Olive observed that 'the pupils that...have had to change carers at the age of sixteen, things have gone drastically wrong for, very, very quickly'. Ms Lea referred to a 'flashpoint', when 'all of a sudden all our really good kids don't want to go to school anymore', and Ms Teal observed 'very often...Year 11 [age 15–16] is destined to be a nightmare...it's awful, sometimes...December onwards...you sort of watch it unravel'. Professionals spoke of advocating for placement continuity post-16:

> I fight very hard...I get really quite arsey...even if they became eighteen at the beginning of Year 13...it's now accepted I think that they will stay in that placement until they've finished their education, so 'til they leave school (Ms Ford).

Niall's case provides a striking example of the importance of continuity as young people transition in education and care at age 16. Although Ms Carmine did not consider Niall's carer to be adequate, she nonetheless thought that it would better for him to remain with her as he made the transition to college at 16, because 'he's been through so much, and is still lacking so much confidence, and he still needs so much support, that it would be best that he stays where he is until eighteen, definitely'. She had also endeavoured to arrange for him to continue at her school two days a week when he started college, saying:

> If he doesn't have it, everything that he's worked for in the last year, being here, is really going to be a waste of time, so I'm hoping that they will go for the two days, two mornings, something, that he's still got this connection, where his confidence is building up, he's a lot calmer, he's got a clear focus of where he wants to be, and he's experienced success… if that doesn't happen, yeah, I'll be definitely worried, with regards to his outlook. As of September…he won't last a term.

Unfortunately, the local authority Special Educational Needs service declined to fund the ongoing provision at Ms Carmine's school, and his carer lost her registration status. As Ms Carmine prophesied, in the absence of ongoing pastoral support from the school, Niall's transition to college failed. He was excluded from college early in the first term, disrupted a second college placement and remained NEET thereafter.

Disruption was particularly acute where young people were moved back into their local authorities from out-of-area placements at 16, for example where therapeutic residential care homes only cared for younger children (Mr Steel) or consequent upon resource issues (Ms Olive). Some participants described young people placed out-of-area being told that if they did not achieve the GCSE grades required for sixth form entry, they would be relocated to their home authority to attend college, losing their carer, social worker, school and friends. Such pressure was likely to trigger 'all sorts of anxiety, all sorts of acting out, and all sorts of very challenging behaviour…' (Ms Teal). Both attachment theory and the focal model of adolescence are useful in understanding these reactions and providing insight into young people's experiences more broadly.

Adolescence, attachment and placement disruption

Although security of attachment to parents is associated with more positive behaviour and better emotional regulation in adolescence (Allen et al., 2003; Hershenberg et al., 2011), Van Eijck et al.'s (2012) longitudinal study of over 1,300 adolescents in the general population found that anxiety increases from early to middle adolescence. Poorer perceived attachment relationships with fathers predicted greater General Anxiety Disorder (GAD) symptoms, but adolescent GAD symptoms were a significant predictor of perceived attachment quality in relation to both parents. It is not known whether this latter finding is a result of parental responses to anxiety in adolescents or the effect of anxiety on adolescents' perceptions of their relationships with parents (van Eijck et al., 2012). In relation to children in care, this might mean that while attachment problems in birth parent relationships are implicated in the development of anxiety symptoms in adolescence, those symptoms may in turn impact on the quality of the attachment relationship with foster carers. Further, loss of an established care-giving relationship coupled with extensive disruption in other domains of their lives may be particularly problematic in mid-adolescence when anxiety increases and relationships with new carers may be more difficult to establish.

Attention to attachment style in adolescence is important for children in care. Empirical evidence of the influence of maltreated children's attachment style to birth parents on subsequent relationships in adolescence is limited, but research suggests that children with insecure attachment to birth parents can develop secure attachments to foster carers. Despite evidence of genetic influence on attachment style in adolescents from relatively advantaged backgrounds (Fearon et al., 2014), in foster children, placement duration and positive maternal behavioural interactions correlate strongly to security of attachment to foster mother (Joseph et al., 2014). Joseph et al. compared 62 children aged 10–17 in foster care with 50 peers matched as a group for age, gender and ethnicity who had lived with at least one birth parent throughout their life. Although the foster care group displayed considerably greater behavioural difficulties than the comparison group, adolescents with a secure attachment to foster carers were reported by carers as displaying fewer Callous-Unemotional traits as measured by the Antisocial Process Screening Device Callous–Unemotional scale and fewer conduct problems on the Strengths and Difficulties Questionnaire. The authors draw attention to the significance of this finding in the context of the known association between disruptive behaviour and placement breakdown and the longer-term risk of a pattern of 'placement careers' (van Santen, 2015).

Resolution of attachment difficulties is also important for young people's mental and emotional health. For example, maternal attachment anxiety in early adolescence is related to greater reported difficulty in adjusting to relationship loss, including bereavement (Fagundes et al., 2012), an issue for all children removed from parental care. Self-harm in early adulthood is strongly associated with disorganised attachment (Stroufe, 2005). Adolescents who have suffered violence exhibit higher rates of mental health problems. Concurrent multiple negative life events also increase vulnerability to mental illness, but young people experiencing both negative life events and insecure attachment are at greater risk of mental ill health than would be expected from the sum of the two risk effects individually (Bannink et al., 2013). This suggests that secure attachment in adolescence may offer a protective factor to buffer the impact of life events on adolescents' mental health (Bannink et al., 2013). Attachment state of mind in early adolescence also appears to be important for young people's ability to make supportive romantic relationships and manage conflicts in those relationships (Tan et al., 2016), with insecurity in parental and peer attachment in adolescence predicting a more anxious style of attachment in romantic relationships in adulthood (Pascuzzo et al., 2013). These findings may have particular implications for young people likely to move to live independently at a relatively early age.

Insights into young people's experiences from the focal model of adolescence

In this study eight young people entered care (or at least were removed from the care of their parents) before the start of secondary school. Within this group are all six of the young people with the most stable placements (Adam, Imogen, Jacinda, Kayla, Michael and Tasmin), of which all but Michael (who had special educational needs) were amongst the young people with the highest educational qualifications and the most likely to progress to university. Five of the participants entered care aged 13 or over (Niall, Priya, Qadira, Riley and Sofia), and, with the exception of the unaccompanied asylum-seeker Sofia, whose situation was unknown, this group were all NEET at the end of the study. High-achieving late entrants comprised only the two orphans, Bashir and Devora.

This study sample therefore reflects the wider picture of poorer outcomes associated with late entrance into care (Sinclair et al., 2007). The accounts given by both young people and professionals to explain their difficulties resonate with the focal model in the way in which young people may struggle to engage in education when they face concurrent issues in their personal lives. These include Adam, who was unable to focus on academic performance in his first few years in care, the young man described by Ms Tan as abandoning schoolwork when reintroduced to his mother and Priya, who stressed her need to 'sort her life out' before she could address education. While treatment or counselling for trauma may be required before some young people can move on in their lives, the focal model helps to explain more broadly why the 'accelerated and compressed' transitions to adulthood (Stein, 2006a: 174) so often experienced by care leavers, particularly those entering care late, may be unmanageable for them. From the perspective of the focal model, state education and social care institutions are organised in such a way as to superimpose social transitions, such as the move to the leaving care team and progression from school to college, upon naturally occurring developmental tasks for young people who are already facing a backlog of deficits in education. This is arguably an example of the way in which institutions may operate, albeit unwittingly, to reproduce power or disadvantage as described by Fineman (2008). In this context, we should be unsurprised by professional accounts of young people's lives 'unravelling' as Ms Teal described it, in the period under consideration in this study. But the focal model is primarily concerned with the developmental *relationship* demands of adolescence, and the following section considers the contribution of the focal model in explaining young people's preoccupation with and renegotiation of birth family relationships as they aged out of care.

Renegotiating birth family relationships

As discussed in Chapter 2, one of the key developmental tasks of adolescence is construction of a theory of the self. Although peers become more influential in young people's lives in adolescence, parents remain the most important source of support in the development of self-concept (Call and Mortimer, 2001), and the significance of parental support to self-esteem, a key aspect of self-concept, does not decline and remains critical in the domains of school and family (Harter, 2012). The concept of 'arenas of comfort' (Simmons et al., 1987) suggests that stability of positive birth family contact may go some way to mitigate the stress of multiple concurrent life changes, but as recounted in Chapter 3, this was more often a cause of considerable distress for participants. For young people in care, late adolescence brings the opportunity to renegotiate these relationships, often after lengthy periods in which they have been constrained or managed by children's social care services. Participants to this study were highly preoccupied with their relationships with their birth families, but as they grew older, they tended to take greater responsibility for managing them.

Kayla's response is a good example of young people's replies when asked what their priorities were in the final interview: 'right now, I'm getting to know the rest of my family'. Kayla managed these family relationships with responsibility and care. She saw her sister 'quite frequently' but explained in her third interview:

> I haven't seen her this month. I did it on purpose because…since I…was eighteen, I've seen her so much. And it's like I have other people to see as well, and she can't just depend on me to just see her. So I just like make sure that she knows I'm here…I can come see her occasionally, not every week…I really go to see my sister to see my nieces, that's important.

When asked whether she saw the importance of these relationships as primarily for her benefit or that of her family, Kayla replied:

> It's more important for me to know that I have that link with them, but they also feel an importance that I have the link with them, because they think I'm a positive role model, which I can say I think I am, for my nieces anyway.

Riley had set fire to the family home and been remanded into care after his family 'washed their hands' of him. He rated his birth family as probably the most important people in his life and had invested a lot of effort in repairing the relationship with his mother, including making a two-hour train journey each weekend to visit. However, he presented as remarkably self-contained and managed the relationship with his family carefully: 'Never really tell them much…They just know what they need to know'. Like Riley, Bashir ensured he kept in contact with his family ('what I've got left of') and that he called his grandfather in Pakistan from his uncle's house 'because he worries about us, obviously'. Callum expressed guilt at having neglected his birth family while setting up his new flat in his third interview:

> I've just really been focusing on myself at the moment, just to get stuff sorted out for the flat and looking after myself, but this week I'm going to see quite a lot of the family...I ain't seen my mum in about two months. I feel bad for that. Christmas as well, I haven't seen her, feel really bad.

For some young people, attaining 18 enabled them to forge re-establish relationships with members of their birth family they had previously been prohibited from seeing. This opportunity may provide a 'turning point' (Masten et al., 2004) in young people's lives or become a significant distraction from other issues, such as their education. Niall's mother, according to his social worker, had 'completely abandoned him it seems'. Towards the end of the project, Niall had got back in touch with his mother – but his social worker considered he was 'finding that hard to process': he was by then unemployed.

Devora was intending to seek information from the court to trace her maternal grandparents, of whose existence she had been unaware until her cousin had found some papers. She explained that on her mother's death, her grandparents had wanted to be involved in her life but her father had cut them out completely, going so far as to tell Devora that her mother had been an orphan: 'I don't know any of my mum's side...I mean I don't even know what my mum looked like.' Kayla, despite having previously chosen not to see her mother, reinstituted contact and visited her for her birthday, but the relationship was not that of parent to child: 'she's just like a friend to me now, she's always got young girls at [the] house who are my age, I don't mind, I just chill with the girls...I'm used to it now.'

Assessing young people's resilient adaptation

There are obvious parallels between aspects of the focal model of adolescence and a resilience framework. For example, the notion in the resilience literature that the clustering of risk factors reduces the likelihood of resilient adaptation resonates with the proposition in the focal model that young people address challenges consecutively and may not be able to manage concurrent multiple life changes. Both theories have been used in this analysis because they offer different insights into the particular experiences of young people ageing out of care. As explained above, the focal model is of particular relevance because it is premised upon the developmental context of adolescence. Resilient adaptation in contrast is pertinent to, and may change over, the life course and may be influenced in unpredictable ways by critical events (MacDonald, 2007). However, it is the framework most commonly used to consider the trajectories of care leavers, doubtless because as a co-hort they experience higher exposure to the identified risk factors for poor resilient adaptation (Coleman and Hagell, 2007). Strengths of a resilience framework also include acknowledgement of children's agency, incorpora-tion of the effect of interaction between the child and their environment and a focus on strengths and competence rather than deficits and maladjustment (Luthar and Cicchetti, 2000).

A resilience framework was chosen for the CLET study for two reasons. First, evidence indicates that educational attainment is a key factor in facilitating resilient adaptation in adolescence, together with a supportive relationship with a competent adult, a sense of personal agency and good peer relationships (Masten et al., 1990; Luthar and Cicchetti, 2000; Rutter, 2000). Second, Stein (2012) has developed a categorisation of care leavers based on the principles of resilient adaptation (set out in Chapter 4). This is adopted in the following analysis in relation to the young people from the CLET study. It is important to bear in mind that this analysis is made tentatively and in acknowledgement that participants were still very young at the time the study ended, with considerable uncertainty and fluidity in all aspects of their lives. Nonetheless the exercise is arguably a useful one in assessing the likely life trajectories of young people in early adulthood and is used to inform the application of foundational rights theory to young people's experiences in the following chapter, from which implications for the attention of policy-makers are drawn.

Applying Stein's categorisations to young people's experiences

In Tables 7.2–7.4 young people are organised into suggested categories (Stein, 2006b; Stein, 2012) on the basis of their history and circumstances at the end of the study, in so far as they were known. The typical charac-teristics of each group are stated in an abbreviated fashion below for ease of reference (a fuller account of the categories is given in Chapter 4). Young people are given one to three stars (★) to indicate their apparent functioning in each domain: to an extent the judgement is inevitably influenced by my impressions of young people in interview. Ollie is not included, as he will be dependent all his life, but it should be noted that there is a dearth of liter-ature on the experiences and outcomes of disabled care leavers, who are at greater risk of ongoing discrimination, bullying and maltreatment in young adulthood (Kelly et al., 2016).

Moving on: Stability; secure attachment; some educational success; left care later than average in a planned move; felt well-prepared for independence; able to take advantage of support; positive identity through participating in the 'normal' trajectories of further or higher education, partnering and parenthood.

Survivors: Regard themselves as self-reliant but often continue to depend on services and have difficulty making and keeping supportive relation-ships; left care younger, often in response to a trigger incident; limited or no academic qualifications; may be assisted by new supportive relationships and stable accommodation; rekindling birth family relationships may be helpful or problematic.

Strugglers: Pre-care maltreatment militates against stability in care; cumulative histories of disruption and emotional, behavioural and social problems may culminate in rejection and alienation of professional and personal support; early age of leaving care; a high likelihood of unemployment and homelessness requiring specialist professional services.

The wide range of young people's life trajectories can be seen clearly from Tables 7.2–7.4. Excluding Ollie, there are 20 young people, of whom nine appear to be moving on, five surviving, one struggling (Niall) and five categorised as surviving/struggling. The numbers are too small to be regarded as representative of the population and will have been influenced by the way in which young people were accessed: that is, through designated teachers in the main, but through a specialist leaving care support charity in the case of three vulnerable young people (Priya, Qadira and Unity). However, it is worth noting that the proportion of young people 'Moving On' is higher than that expected from Stein's work and that these young people appear to be well-placed academically to succeed in adulthood. Five (Adam, Bashir, Jacinda, Kayla and Tasmin) were expected to attain the qualifications needed to attend university, although it is likely that only Kayla, Tasmin and Adam would do so in the year they left school, as Bashir did not obtain any offers to study Medicine and was reluctant to take the alternative course for which he had a place. Adam would take an apprenticeship instead of a university place if he could obtain one, and Jacinda was a year behind her peers after transferring to college at 17. Tasmin was not interviewed in her final year at school. Devora had good GCSE results but had chosen to progress to a performing arts BTEC (vocational) qualification at college.

The three girls in the 'university' group plus Devora were the four participants with the most stable and supportive relationships with a key adult in their lives, in Devora's case her cousin and for the remaining three their foster carer. Adam and Bashir had also described supportive and stable foster care, despite choosing to leave for independent accommodation at the age of 18. All six exhibited a strong sense of personal agency and all reported good peer relationships, although Kayla was cautious and selective in her choice of friends, and Devora had felt friendless at school but had made good relationships at college. It would have been useful to have been able to follow these young people for another year after they left school or college, in particular to ask for their views on their accommodation choices in hindsight.

The three remaining young people categorised as 'Moving On' were Imogen, Michael and Sofia. Relatively little data were gathered from Michael and Sofia, both of whom participated in the study only once. Michael had Asperger's Syndrome and rarely answered the questions asked, instead choosing his own agenda for the conversation. He was in a stable placement with his sister, where he had been since the age of four, and was successfully

Table 7.2 Summary of young people's risk and protective factors using Stein's resilience categorisations: 'moving on'

Name	Stability	Educational success	Planned/early exit	Prepared for independence	Supportive relationships	Positive identity
Adam	★★ From end of primary school	★★★ University offers	★★ Can stay with carers but chooses to leave at 18	★★★ Working, well-supported, mature	★★ With carers, DT, SW, not birth family	Self-reliant but readily accepts help, good peer relationships
Bashir	★★ Since entry to UK age 12/13	★★★ Predicted 4 A*s at A2	★★ Can stay with carers but chooses to leave at 18	★★★ Mature and self-sufficient, extended family in UK	★★ With carers, extended family – lost birth family	Self-reliant, hard-working and ambitious
Devora	★★★ With cousin since care at age 13	★★★ Good GCSEs, then BTEC, struggling to get perf. arts place	★★ Can stay with carer but chooses to leave at 18	★★ Mature and reflective	★★ Especially with cousin (carer)	Responsible, empathetic, sees herself as orphan rather than LAC
Imogen	★ 'Loads' of carers, unhappy in long-term placement	★★ Modest but steady progress	● Sudden disruption in year 12	★★★ Managing supported independent accommodation well	★★ Poor relationship with carer, good with birth M and extended foster family	Very quiet, appears timid but thoughtful
Jacinda	★★ At least four placements, stable from age eight – feels like own family	★ To college at 17 after struggling at school, planning university (Nursing)	★★★ Expects to stay put until graduates	★★★ Able to take her time, proactive in seeking educational support	★★ Excellent relationship with foster carers, problematic with birth family	Seems somewhat lacking in confidence at times
Kayla	★★★ Two carers, last from age six	★★★ Expecting to go to university (Sports Psychology /Coaching)	★★★ Expects to stay put until first university long vacation	★★★ Able to take her time, proactive in seeking educational support	★ Good relationship with carers, complex with birth family	Difficulty with personal relationships, otherwise good; many extracurricular activities
Michael	★★★ From age four	★★? (Asperger's Syndrome)	★★★ Carers would have liked to adopt	★★★ Able to take his time (young for age)	★★ Good relationship with carers, but slightly anxious	Confident
Sofia?	★ To UK age 16, short placement	?	★★? Chose semi-independent at 18	? Mature but limited English	? Difficulty making peer relationships	Mature and highly self-reliant
Tasmin	★★★ Four carers, last since Y9 (age 13/14)	★★ Planning to go to university	★★ Placement pressure: brother's behaviour	★★ Mature and well-supported	★★ Excellent relationship with carer	Strong and lively character

Table 7.3 Summary of young people's risk and protective factors using Stein's resilience categorisations: 'survivors'

Name	Stability	Educational success	Planned exit	Prepared for independence	Supportive relationships	Positive identity
Elliott	★★ Stable foster care 11–16, then unknown	Dropped out of college at 16/17 NEET	Unknown–wanted to live with birth family at 16	?	★★ With carers, extended family – none with birth family	Wanted to be footballer or join fire service
Farouk	★ Two placements, 1st unhappy, stable from end Y9 (age 14)	Mostly Ds at GSCE, excluded from college (imm) Y12, back in education Y13	★★ Could have stayed with carers but left to live with brother at 18	★ Carers protective, brother struggling to engage in education	★ Ex-carers supportive, brother unlikely to be positive role model	Anxious about immigration, fitness and being out of education in 2nd interview
Habib	Four carers from age nine, last one for four to five years	★ Excluded from school; PRU; repeating level 1 college Y13	💣 Sudden disruption	★ Supported independent accommodation clean and tidy but bare; struggling with college attendance	Felt rejected by carers and that they treated own son differently	Making concrete plans for future
Luis	In care at seven, stable from age nine	★ Excluded, SEBD school, limited quals but attending college in 2nd interview	★★ Expects to stay with carers post-18 as younger sister there	Will need ongoing adult services	None apparent, with possible exception of older brother	Confused aspirations
Riley (Moving on if not NEET)	Youth justice route into care, two res homes	★ PRU, College level 2 Public Services, dropped out NEET	★ Residential care ended at 16, to supported lodgings	★★ Self-reliant and competent, retaking army medical technician exams	★ Good relationship with landlords (supported lodgings), manages birth family and peers	Articulate and frank, clear-sighted and personable, clear (but changeable?) plans for the future

Table 7.4 Summary of young people's risk and protective factors using Stein's resilience categorisations: 'survivors/strugglers' and 'strugglers'

Name	Stability	Educational success	Planned/ early exit	Prepared for independence	Supportive relationships	Positive identity
Callum **survivor/ struggler**	Disrupted care history, difficult to care for	★ Few quals, hopes to stay extra year at school	●✱ Sudden disruption age 16/17	★ Lonely living independently but seems to be coping	★ With designated teacher, girlfriend	Little idea what he would like to do
Gilroy **survivor/ struggler**	★ Single placement from entry to care age 11/12 but broke down when 16/17	Poor KS4 quals, 'kicked out' of college age 16/17, about to start '18' project **NEET**	●✱ Sudden disruption age c16	★ In semi-independent at 16 but appeared unsettled	Unhappy in care, no strong relationship mentioned	Lacks confidence and maturity (Ms White), desire to go to university, 'too old' to be footballer
Priya **survivor/ struggler**	Foster care from age 13, four care homes from age 15	Left school at 16, seemingly no quals, college briefly, **NEET**	Move to supported accommodation at 16 – claims averse to living with strangers	Managing in supported accommodation with intensive keyworker support, tends not to attend for interviews etc.	Struggles to engage with professionals, avoids relationships with men, spends a lot of time with mother	Feels unable to engage in education until has 'sorted out' her life
Qadira **survivor/ struggler**	In care at age 12/13, three carers	Left school age 14/15. NVQ level 1 hair dressing and literacy **NEET**	Move to supported accommodation at 16	Managing in supported accommodation with intensive keyworker support	None apparent apart from key worker	Looking for jobs/ trying to get on track to go to college
Unity **survivor/ struggler**	Strong history of placement disruption – c10 res homes	Did not really attend secondary school, reluctant to go to college **NEET**	Move to supported accommodation at 16	Managing in supported accommodation with intensive keyworker support	Difficult relationships with professionals, lost touch with supporting charity at 18	Angry at move away from home area
Niall **Struggler**	Into care 12/13, four carers, last 'on and off'	Not literate, Excluded schools and colleges **NEET**	Carer lost status when 16/17	Semi-independent, did not attend housing panel	Not engaging at 17/18	Social worker third year of study: finding it hard to process renewal of relationship with his mother

attending a mainstream school. His carers would have adopted him had it not been for the fact that they would then have lost the social care support they received. Sofia spoke little about her personal life and had not been in the UK long when we spoke; she struggled to make friends in school, perhaps because she was a year below her chronological age but mature for her years as a result of her personal history, as well as because of her limited English. However, she was articulate and determined, had a strong sense of agency and appeared to be making good progress academically in the short space of time since she had arrived in the UK.

Imogen was a quiet but thoughtful young woman whose designated teacher was concerned that she would not cope at college and thought she should remain at school post-16. Imogen chose to go to college 'to make a new start', and contrary to Ms Gold's expectations, progressed well there and was on track at the end of the study to become a nursery teacher. Imogen had had a difficult relationship with her foster mother from around the age of 10 until the placement broke down when she was 17. She confided her unhappiness in the placement only to a peer who was a member of her foster carer's extended family, with whom she had good relationships. She did not feel able to tell any adult at school or any of her social workers. Imogen returned briefly to her birth mother on being forced to leave her foster home (before being provided with her own accommodation) and felt that she should never have been placed in care, although she acknowledged that it had been beneficial in terms of educational support.

A high proportion of the young participants faced significant uncertainty at the end of the study, not least the seven young people who were NEET, namely Elliott, Gilroy, Niall, Priya, Qadira, Riley and Unity. The social worker of one of these young people described them in the final year of the study as very angry, 'gang-affiliated', friendless apart from a dog, and with rotten teeth. The remaining four young people (Callum, Farouk, Habib and Luis) were in school or college but had limited qualifications and uncertain prospects. Nine of these 11 young people were living in independent or semi-independent accommodation (including Riley, in supported lodgings); Elliott's placement status was unknown, and Luis remained in foster care with his younger sister, but would require adult social care services. The less settled and academically successful young people in the study tended to be less forthcoming or less articulate in interview, so it was more difficult to assess aspects of resilient adaptation such as their sense of personal agency and good peer relationships. However, seven of these 11 young people experienced placement breakdowns during or shortly before the start of the study, and eight had been excluded from school or college or dropped out. Six of the young people (Gilroy, Habib, Niall, Priya, Qadira and Unity) had suffered recent disruption in both care and educational domains. Only Farouk maintained stability in care and education – and he chose to leave his placement to live with his brother at 18 and missed the first year of further education as a result of exclusion from college because of his immigration status. Callum had a very difficult placement history and was fortunate to have been able to remain in a supportive school environment where the designated teacher had provided a stable and supportive adult figure in a pastoral role throughout Callum's secondary schooling.

The literature suggests that young women may be more likely to achieve better outcomes from care and more resilient adaptations generally (McGloin and Widom, 2001; Jackson and Ajayi, 2007). Although the participant group comprised 12 young men and nine young women, six of the nine classified as 'Moving On' were young women, and the remaining three young women were accessed through a specialist charity providing supported housing to care leavers from 16 to 18. Only three of the young men appeared to be well-placed to progress to independence, and it is possible that Michael's Asperger's Syndrome might require ongoing support into adulthood, leaving only Adam and Bashir in this group.

When asked who knew about their care status in school, four of the girls (Imogen, Jacinda, Kayla and Tasmin) all referred to 'best' or 'close' friends, indicating strong close peer relationships. Four girls (Devora, Jacinda, Kayla and Tasmin) were also the young people with the closest relationships with their carers. In interview, the young women tended to be better able to explain their motivations and feelings and on the whole appeared more mature. However, the four girls in the first group above all entered care while of primary-school age, and the girls as a whole fell into three clear groups: early entrants (Moving On), comprising Imogen, Jacinda, Kayla and Tasmin; late entrants (Surviving/Struggling), made up of Priya, Qadira and Unity; and those with no one holding parental responsibility (Moving On), namely Devora and Sofia.

In respect of the young men, the picture is more complex. The two young men who entered care aged 13 or over (Niall and Riley) were both NEET and categorised as Struggling and Surviving respectively. Of the two, Riley exhibited a much greater sense of agency, with clear plans for the future, including contingency arrangements, and seemingly a stable and supportive, if somewhat short-term, relationship with his landlords. Four of the young men entered care in the first two years of secondary school (Bashir, Callum, Farouk and Gilroy), of whom Gilroy was NEET at the end of the study and only Bashir is classified as Moving On. The remaining five (Adam, Elliott, Habib, Luis and Michael, as well as Ollie) entered care before reaching secondary school age, but of these, only Adam and Michael are classified as Moving On, and Elliott dropped out of college and became NEET. Of the three refugee or asylum-seeking young men, Bashir was doing well, but Farouk had left his carers, and Habib's placement had broken down. Farouk and Habib both had limited academic qualifications.

Black and ethnic minority young people were over-represented in the group, of whom nine were White, four Asian, three Black, and four mixed race (Black), with one (Luis) mixed race (other). However, there has been no discernible pattern in outcomes to date by ethnicity, with the Moving

On group comprising four White young people, one Asian, two Black and two mixed race. The three most vulnerable girls (Priya, Qadira and Unity) were Asian, Black, and White respectively and the young men most at risk of social exclusion were Niall (White) and probably Callum (White). This may support the contention that Fineman's analysis of the way in which institutions may operate to reproduce power or disadvantage (Fineman, 2008) might in some respects be a more fruitful approach in seeking to understand care leavers' life trajectories than a focus on young people's individual characteristics such as ethnicity, particularly in contexts where racial and ethnic backgrounds are becoming increasingly diverse.

One of the key factors in Stein's categorisation relates to the notion of self-reliance: young people able to take advantage of support available in and on leaving care are likely to be Moving On; Survivors tend to regard themselves as self-reliant; while Strugglers are alienated from or by professional support. The way in which aspects of the care 'system' tend to operate to promote or enhance the development of self-reliance has been discussed in Chapter 4, but there are two issues related to this that stood out in the CLET study, which may be related to one another and which deserve more detailed consideration. The first of these is the nature and availability of adult support from young people's perspectives and the second is the tendency for young people to reject the opportunity to remain in foster placements once they left school or turned 18, in favour of living independently.

Self-reliance and supportive adult relationships

Chapter 4 included a brief review of the coping and resilience literature concerned with the crucial role of social support, including evidence that, for adolescents, the family plays the most important role in buffering young people from stress (Seiffge-Krenke, 1995; Coleman, 2011). For the majority of children in care (possibly excluding UASC), their birth family is a source of stress rather than of its alleviation, explaining the particular importance of substitute caring adult relationships in their lives, as highlighted by researchers such as Schofield (2001) and Geenen and Powers (2007). Parental responsibility for children in care vests in a corporation, but there are four potential sources of stable supportive adult relationships for this group: foster carers (or staff in residential accommodation), social workers, teachers and informal acquaintances.

Smith, in a reevaluation of residential child care, not only highlights the centrality of adult–child relationships in children's care but distinguishes relationships with children made by other professionals (such as doctors and teachers) from those made by residential child care workers by virtue of the fact that only for professionals in care settings is the primary task the building of relationships with children (Smith, 2009). This distinction helps explain why teachers from mainstream schools in this study, with the exception of Mr Brown, were not regarded by young people as adults with whom they could build close, trusting relationships. This finding should not in any sense be regarded as a criticism of teaching staff. In recent years schools have been seen as a forum in which many of the ills of society can be remedied, in particular those that stem from poor or disadvantaged parenting. Concurrently, however, there has been an increased focus on raising academic attainment through managerial systems of monitoring and assessment (Gewirtz, 2002). Schools remain hierarchical establishments primarily concerned with educational outcomes. The advantages of the designated teacher post, and of its holder being a senior member of staff, have already been outlined, but such a role is unlikely to be compatible with the relationship-based practice of traditional care work. However, Smith also bemoans the extent to which the centrality of the worker–client relationship in social work has been replaced by outcomes-driven case management approaches, concluding that '[c]are only becomes meaningful when it is personal' (121). A return to relationship-based practice in English child protection social work has also been called for by Lonne et al. (2009) and Munro (2011), amongst others.

With the exception of Adam, none of the young people in this study reported close personal relationships with their social workers, as explored in Chapter 4. For the most part, social worker turnover precluded social workers being able to afford consistent supportive guidance to young people within a personal adult–child relationship. There was some evidence that key workers or personal advisers fared better in making meaningful relationships with young people, but in all cases these were short-lived (generally, at most, from age 16 to 18). Although young people drew on informal relationships such as mentors and non-academic or administrative staff in schools, these appeared primarily to be used in order to contain information about their care status and to avoid the appearance of difference. None of the young people in this study highlighted strong and supportive personal relationships with non-professional adults other than carers, although Ms Olive commented that boys at her school often made strong relationships with their taxi drivers because they saw them every day. Smith (2009: 142) considers that many agencies appear to 'actively discourage the establishment of such relationships', a state of affairs that he points out is exacerbated by highly regulated access to children by adults.

Foster carers are the adults in young people's lives who approximate most closely to parental role models and are best placed to provide the supportive adult relationship described above. The correlation between stable, supportive placements and successful outcomes for young people has already been discussed and it is deplorable that so few participants reported being treated as a member of the foster carer's family. Urgent attention needs to be given to the recruitment, training and retention of good quality foster carers, including those qualified and able to work with children with complex needs, and to ensure that foster carers are adequately supported in their role (Colton et al., 2008; Randle et al., 2016). Calls for professionalisation of the role should be considered (Randle et al., 2016), but such action may have significant implications for the development of caring parent–child relationships. As Ms Tan said of the children in her school:

> you want them to have caring adults around them who will care for them until they are nineteen, and twenty-five, and thirty, who will be there for them, just like my family was there for me all my life. And they are a rare commodity, finding foster carers who will say I've taken on this child, I will not give up on this child no matter how unbearable they become...It is a job and you get paid for it, but it's not a job.

This insight perhaps contributes to explaining the evidence from this study that young people were likely to reject the opportunity to remain in foster placements in favour of living independently, considered in the following section.

Leaving care

Opting for independence

Living independently appeared to become more attractive to participants as they aged through the study. This finding applied to some of the young people in successful, stable placements as well as to those who were less settled. Legislation to allow more young people to remain in their foster placements until the age of 21 came into force shortly after the conclusion of the study (Children and Families Act 2014 s98). Local authorities must now consider the appropriateness of the child 'staying put' with their foster carer at the time of preparation of the pathway plan (that is, ideally soon after the child reaches 16); they must facilitate such an arrangement if both parties wish it, and it is 'appropriate'; and they must support the arrangement until the young person is 21, including through financial support to the former foster carer, unless they consider that the arrangement is not consistent with the young person's welfare. In Scotland, since 2015, the Children and Young People (Scotland) Act 2014 has offered young people the option to remain in their care placement, whether foster, kinship or residential, to the age of 21. The changes were based on a pilot scheme (Munro et al., 2012), as well as evidence from the US on the economic benefits of allowing young people to remain in foster care longer (Peter et al., 2009). Initial indications suggest that this initiative has had modest success; government statistics for England

(DfE/NS, 2016a) show a slight fall in 19-year-old care leavers living independently from 40 per cent in 2015 to 37 per cent in 2016 and a rise from four to six per cent in those 'staying put' with foster carers.

In the CLET study, however, a surprising number of participants presented themselves as actively choosing independence, even where they described a good relationship with their carers and could have stayed beyond the age of 18. In a study of young people aged 18–25 ageing out of care in the US, Pryce et al. (2017) observed a similar reluctance to remain in foster care beyond the age of 18, reflecting a desire to move on from dependence on the care system into independent adulthood and entrenched habits of self-reliance. The initiative and self-reliance exhibited by young people as well as the nature of the relationship with carers may go some way to explaining these choices among the CLET cohort. Bashir, for example, despite stating initially that he treated his foster carers like his new parents when he came to the UK because he knew he had lost his family, explained:

> I wouldn't prefer to stay with my carer. I want to be more independent…I've made roots with them, but not…as strong as if it was my own parents, obviously. I'll be leaving when I'm eighteen, but I'm still going to be in contact with them…because they've helped us quite a lot.

Adam, too, decided not to remain with his carers. In his first interview he had said that although social services would pay his carer only until he reached 18, 'my carer said because she's so nice I can stay with her until I want'. But in the final year of the study he was planning to move, explaining 'I'd rather have the accommodation…I just think it's better to get on the ladder early, instead of late', although he thought it 'might be a bit scary at first'. Devora did not want to leave her cousin but was conscious that she was a significant drain on her finances ('now that I've turned eighteen my guardian isn't getting any funding'), and her carer had advised Devora to get on the housing ladder, too. Imogen said she could have stayed with her birth mother when her foster mother excluded her from her home but did not because she liked the idea of having her own flat. She said 'I love living on my own. I don't have people saying [Imogen] can you do this, [Imogen] can you do that'. Riley could have stayed in his supported lodgings until he was 21, but although he had a good relationship with his landlords he wanted 'to move out soon', partially because there was another young man there who had arrived after him, who kept disappearing, stealing and damaging things. Farouk chose to leave his carers to live with his brother when he reached 18, and Priya reported that her aversion to living with strangers had eventually prompted social services to allow her to live in supported accommodation on her own.

Anxieties

The choice to opt for independent accommodation was made by young people despite their acute awareness of the financial and practical pressures they were likely to experience as a consequence:

> if you are living with your own parents and stuff it's obviously much more easier for you to kind of just concentrate on your studies and other things in your life as well (Bashir).
>
> I'm just worried if I can't get a job in the future, you know (Callum).

Adam was working 11 hours a day on Saturdays and Sundays in the final year of the study ('it's just I need to get some more money to have behind me'), but he would have to give up his job once he had a flat or his income support would be greatly reduced. Bashir was intending to work over the summer because he had been advised that his budget would be 'very tight' when he lived independently. Tasmin's carer had set her the task of living on £50 a week and was refusing to cook for her, to persuade her she should stay in foster care rather than move to live with her sister:

> just to prove that I couldn't do it. So I am gonna prove her wrong... I'm starting it tomorrow. I'm really scared about it. I'm dreading it. So everything's so expensive, all my food, because of everything I'm allergic to, so costs so much money.

Other young people had not chosen to live independently. Callum was pleased and proud to be placed with his aunt and uncle during the first year of the study. In the second interview, he concluded that he would prefer to stay with his aunt and uncle than live independently:

> my carer is my auntie, she's family, so it wouldn't be a problem anyway [to stay]...I won't be moving as soon as I'm eighteen, I want to stay for quite a while...Yeah, I don't want to move because it's my auntie and my uncle, and they are still my carers but they are my auntie and uncle.

Unfortunately, the placement broke down and by the final interview Callum was living independently. Callum, who had a history of criminal violence, was daunted by the prospect of living alone:

> I didn't want to move because I didn't think I could handle it. You know, at first I couldn't really handle it, living by myself, but now I can...My girlfriend, yeah, she helps a lot. Sometimes it does get very lonely as well, and she comes around, keeps me company, and she'll bring a couple of my friends as well...I mean at first I wasn't really comfortable, every little noise I would hear I would get scared. Living by myself I

would just get really paranoid. Yeah, I would just get very lonely, but now, I'm used to it now, I'm *getting* used to it now.

Devora too, was worried:

I actually had a housing interview on Tuesday and they said I'm gonna move out...because I'm eighteen now, and my guardian...thinks that I'm old enough to move out.
How do you feel about that?
Scared.

Adam, having dealt with his sense of rejection by his birth family by deciding to have no more to do with them, was concerned that he would be moved back near his birth family:

it's gonna be weird moving from this area which I'm brought up into, all the way back to [X] where all my family are...
And how do you feel about being back in [X]...?
...it's stupid, that's what everyone's saying now, it's not a really good idea. I don't really want to see them but you have no choice, you have to go back to that area.

Of those whose destinations were known, only Jacinda and Kayla, who were particularly close to their foster families, intended or expected to remain in their placements after leaving school or college. Kayla explained her decision in terms of making a gradual transition to independent living:

my carers said I can stay, but if I get into my uni of my choice I'll live in halls of residence anyway, so it means I'm half moving out anyway, and then if I go on to my second year I'll ask my social worker for my flat, so I can just move from my halls of residence to my flat.

Jacinda intended to take her foster carer's advice:

you know you can get a flat when you turn eighteen, but I don't think I'm going to take it until after uni, then I'd get a flat, that's what my mum told me to do. She said that's a better idea instead of struggling.

Accommodation and prospects

Government statistics (DfE/NS, 2016a) include experimental data for accommodation or placement at 18 for children who were in care at 16. Table 7.5 below shows the accommodation of study participants at the end of the study using the government's categories. National data are given for comparison. Elliott is excluded because his placement was unknown after the first year of the study, and for a few young people it is assumed: for example, Tasmin is assumed to have remained with her foster carer until the end of the school year in which she turned 18 although that placement had been under pressure from her brother's behaviour in the previous year.

These figures show that the young people with the most promising future prospects were either likely to move directly from their carers to independence (Adam, Bashir and Devora) or to remain with their carers for some time post-18 (Jacinda, Kayla, Michael and perhaps Tasmin). Of the two remaining young people categorised as 'Moving On', Imogen's placement had broken down at 17, and Sofia's placement history was unclear, but she only arrived in the UK at age 15 or 16. As well as illustrating the tendency of young people in this study to elect to move into independent accommodation rather than remain with their carers post-18, this table suggests that the Staying Put provisions are unlikely to assist those young people already on the edge of social exclusion. Callum, Gilroy, Habib, Imogen, Niall, Priya, Qadira and Unity would not be eligible for Staying Put because their placements broke down before or during the study

Table 7.5 Young people's accommodation status at the end of the study

Accommodation status	Young people	Proportion of group (%)	National data for 18 year-old care leavers SFR41/2016 (%)
Independent/ moving straight to independent at end of study	Callum, Adam, Bashir, Devora	20	16
Semi-independent accommodation at end of study	Habib, Imogen, Niall, Priya, Qadira, Sofia, Unity (all awaiting/ applying for independent accommodation)	35	21
Supported lodgings	Riley (applying for independent accommodation)	5	9
Foster care	Jacinda, Kayla, Luis, Michael, [Tasmin]	25	19
Custody	Gilroy	5	3 (10 for 17 year olds)
Parents/relatives	Farouk (with brother)	5	12
Care home	Ollie	5	5
[Other/emergency/ not in touch/ unknown]		—	[15]

(in Niall's case, this was an informal placement, and his carer's status was eventually revoked).

What is more certain is that the young people most at risk of poor outcomes were in the least stable accommodation. In its current form, the Staying Put initiative is welcome in providing transitional support for care leavers more closely in line with that of their peers but will only be of benefit to young people who are already well-placed to 'move on' in their lives by the time they reach the age of 18. Devora explained that she was in the second band for priority allocation of housing in her local authority, the first being people who are terminally ill and the second care leavers in full-time education. In contrast, Riley, who was NEET, had been waiting months for a house, but he had recently progressed from band D to band C. Habib had been told that his choice of flat would be dependent on his attendance at college because flats in the area he had chosen were popular, and priority was given to those who could demonstrate a need for proximity to the college. While such policies may incentivize some young people to pursue qualifications, they are likely to disadvantage further the least educated, such as Niall, who was still struggling to read and write at 16 and at risk of homelessness at 18. Yet the government rejected the House of Commons Education Committee's (2014) recommendation that the Staying Put provisions be extended to children in residential care homes, although these young people are likely to be amongst the most vulnerable.

Conclusion

Four features stand out in a comparison of the experiences of the research cohort and their peers derived from this study: a dearth of consistent and supportive adult relationships in their lives, the generally poor prospects of the majority of the group, the diversity and polarity of their educational and life trajectories to date and delayed educational progress coinciding with accelerated transitions to independence. The challenges of supporting older children in care to achieve their potential in school and beyond should not be underestimated. Considering the multiple transitions and personal issues facing young people in the light of Coleman's focal model of adolescence contributes to understanding why care leavers may feel overwhelmed by their circumstances and how that affects their educational progress. Neither Gilroy nor Qadira, both late entrants into care, had managed to settle in school: Gilroy thought care had made no difference to his educational prospects on the basis that he had 'never been someone like to sit down for hours and hours and do stuff'. In contrast, it was several years before Adam felt he was able to engage in school, but having entered care while still of primary-school age, he managed to perform well by the time he was 16 and took his GCSEs.

Older children and young people, perhaps because of the complexities of adolescence and of their lives as they reach legal adulthood, are often 'hard to help'. Mr Steel commented:

> you can quite often estimate who is going to end up as a NEET much earlier than we currently do…I think we've got better tracking systems in place…I have got three that look very definitely like NEETs to me, and yes…we are working on those at the moment, and they've worked intensively with two out of the three, to no avail. We are not able to turn them around.

Mr Steel's virtual school had only recently extended its remit to work with young people from 16 to 18, but it is clear that many will need ongoing support into early adulthood. As set out in Chapter 2, in recent decades the transition to adulthood has universally become protracted and more complicated (Furlong, 2009), prompting identification of the stage of 'emerging adulthood' between 18 and 25 (Arnett, 2000). Today's young people live in a daunting world which is changing at a bewildering pace and in which huge inequalities are compounded by a general downward trend in social mobility. This is also an era in which there is a sharp divide between the prospects of graduates with advanced skills and those with poor qualifications, who are likely to find themselves in low-status and precarious jobs with little chance of advancement or long-term security. The limited research on young people from a care background in emerging adulthood endorses the findings of the CLET study in highlighting the need to address relational issues arising from experiences of loss and disruption and focus on building supportive networks, which will enable help-seeking behaviour. It describes young adults as recognising the need for help while feeling reluctant to seek it on the basis that to accept help is both developmentally inappropriate and reflects dependence rather than self-reliance (Pryce et al., 2017). These considerations, coupled with Arnett's conclusion that emerging adulthood has become the predominant period of identity formation for young people, have significant implications for the responsibilities entrusted to care systems, which are considered in the following chapter.

8   Reconceptualizing the state's duties towards the children in its care

Introduction

The evidence of this study confirms that the last 25 years have witnessed some improvement in the educational prospects of children in care in England (Jackson, 2013b). Like the young people in Berridge's study (2017), almost all the young people in this study acknowledged that removal into care had been the right decision for them, and most acknowledged that being in care had improved their life chances. It should be borne in mind that I was unable to take into account variations in young people's innate abilities (a contested and problematic concept in any event). Rather, the views and expectations of young people and professionals have been used as a basis for assessment of the extent to which young people had reached their educational potential by the end of the study.

As recounted in the previous chapters, most if not all of the young people felt that they had not yet fulfilled their educational potential. The reasons for this are complex and varied and have been explored in some detail in the preceding chapters. They include the effects of young people's pre-care experiences, family circumstances and late entry into care; disruption in their personal lives and education when in care; the multitude of challenges faced simultaneously by young people and coinciding with the developmental tasks of adolescence; multiple transitions and physical moves in education and care imposed by state institutions during late adolescence; and the opportunities to reconnect with birth families arising when young people turned 18.

In this chapter I draw together the findings in relation to young people's care and their education and consider the relationship between the two. I address the challenges inherent in the corporate parenting model in meeting the individual needs of children in care and evaluate the role of designated teachers and virtual school heads in improving the educational and life outcomes for care leavers. I draw on notions of 'reparatory' and 'assumed' responsibility (Hollingsworth, 2013a) to justify the imposition of particular duties owed by corporate parents to care leavers. I utilize Hollingsworth's concept of 'foundational rights' (Hollingsworth, 2013b) as a means of establishing what those duties should entail in terms of enabling young people to attain the necessary capacities to exercise what Hollingsworth designates 'full' autonomy. The concept of foundational rights incorporates consideration not only of concrete capabilities such as educational attainment but also of relational aspects of autonomy. It can therefore contribute to an understanding of what young people need in order to be prepared to exercise genuine or 'full' autonomy in adulthood which incorporates recognition of the interdependence of young people's experiences in education and care (Jackson, 2013b), a key consideration arising from the findings of this study.

Using insights from foundational rights to evaluate young people's care outcomes

Despite the deficiencies of the care system, all 17 young people who took part in interviews in the second year of the study were clear that entry into state care had been the right decision for them, with the notable exception of Imogen, who claimed not to understand why she had been removed from her mother's care and did not consider that it had been necessary for her welfare. Devora spoke candidly of the freedom she enjoyed living with her cousin (and which she had been denied when caring for her father) and was grateful for the opportunities she had been given to engage in social and performing arts activities through financial support from the local authority. Kayla described a 'family pattern' of bigotry and lack of ambition and was clear that care had provided her with 'a safe place' in which she had been able to raise her aspirations and learn to communicate and build relationships with others. Riley said care was the 'best thing that could have ever happened, personally', because 'it got me away from my mates, so I wasn't constantly messing about, getting in trouble with the police'. Tasmin thought that if she had not been taken into care she would 'probably be one of them little hood rats that stand in the corner, their hood up, look really intimidating'. For a number of participants, it is likely that entry into care at an earlier age would have reduced the disadvantages they faced upon entry and enhanced their prospects as they approached adulthood. Riley, for example, felt he should have been removed from his parents at 'about ten' rather than 15, before he got too deeply into trouble.

Just over a third of the group appeared to have enjoyed stable and supportive placements (Adam, Bashir, Devora, Jacinda, Kayla, Michel, Ollie and Tasmin). Others had achieved a stable placement (such as Imogen) or support (e.g. Riley) but not both. At least 13 of the cohort were or would be living independently at or shortly after they reached 18. Only four young people (Jacinda, Kayla, Luis and Michael) seemed likely to 'stay put' in their foster placements after the age of 18. In terms of the social assets identified by Fineman (2008), most of the young people had experienced a dearth of supportive foster family relationships and this was not adequately compensated for by stable and positive relationships with social workers. Perhaps partly as a consequence, young people demonstrated a highly developed sense of self-reliance.

There was also a wide range in the extent to which young people appeared to have been provided with opportunities to attain the central human capabilities Nussbaum designates 'Emotions' and 'Affiliation', such as

> [b]eing able to have attachments to things and people outside [them] selves; to love those who love and care for [them];...[n]ot having one's emotional development blighted by fear and anxiety;...[b]eing able to live with and toward others...to engage in various forms of social interaction; [h]aving the social bases of self-respect and nonhumiliation; being able to be treated as a dignified being whose worth is equal to that of others.
>
> (Nussbaum, 2003: 41)

A significant number, notably Callum, Habib, Niall, Priya, Qadira and Unity, presented as particularly vulnerable in their ability to manage their behaviour and to engage with professionals. The previous chapter charted how these most vulnerable young people were most likely to face discrimination in housing, but young people who demonstrated educational success appeared to be accorded preferential treatment by their corporate parents. Some local authorities appeared to provide ongoing qualified social worker support to young people engaging in education but personal advisors to those who were not. Niall's social worker, for example, was about to stop working with him towards the end of the study because the leaving care team covered 16 to 18 year olds: she had only two young people in her case load over the age of 18, and they were both at university. Niall would be transferred to the transitional team, for vulnerable young adults.

For young people with deep-seated problems that have created barriers to their engagement in education and close relationships with their carers, there was arguably something of a policy and/or practice vacuum. The corporate parent, it appeared, accorded greater attention to 'good' children who conform to parental expectations than 'troublesome' children who are less credit to their corporate parent. This notion is resonant of Goldson's description of the '"deserving"–"undeserving" schism' (Goldson, 2002) and Fionda's 'devils and angels' (Fionda, 2005), both in the context of youth justice. This seemed also to be reflected in the study in, for example, the personal attention and advice that virtual heads offered young people applying to university, perhaps influenced by the inclusion of the percentage of entrants to university from care in national statistics. In this context, the concept of foundational rights draws attention to the way in which such policies can serve to inhibit young people's capacity for 'full' (rather than merely legal) autonomy (Hollingsworth, 2013a) through the state's imposition of discriminatory external conditions on those already hampered by poor internal conditions.

The concept of foundational rights can assist in an analysis of the duties corporate parents should owe to the children in their care in a number of ways. First, its incorporation of autonomy as relational enables a holistic analysis of the conditions and capacities required for 'full' autonomy. In the context of children in care, this helps to elucidate the interdependence of care and educational experiences and outcomes in the lives of care leavers and facilitates examination of this interdependence. Second, a foundational rights perspective explains why the most vulnerable young people have the greatest claim to support from their corporate parent and justifies prioritising the needs of those most at risk of failing to attain a fully autonomous adulthood. It thereby exposes policies which tend to reward young people who are doing relatively well as unjust, particularly in the context of the responsibility owed by the state to young people for whose upbringing the state has taken direct responsibility.

It will be recalled from Chapter 2 that the notion of *reparatory* responsibility reflects the state's duty to redress the harm suffered by children before entering care, or indeed through the care system, while that of *assumed* responsibility explains the state's duty to exercise its responsibilities towards the children in its care in the manner of a responsible parent (Hollingsworth, 2013a). Articulation of these duties can draw valuable insights from consideration of the theories underpinning this book in the light of the notion of foundational rights. Resilience theory points to the factors that are likely to assist young people in overcoming the adversity they have experienced, including educational success and the establishment of at least one consistent and caring adult relationship. As considered in the previous chapter, the security of young people's attachment style in adolescence influences their ability to form and maintain mutually supportive romantic relationships in adulthood. The focal model of adolescence explains the need for corporate parents to give young people adequate time to tackle the developmental tasks of adolescence as well as to address the emotional trauma, educational deficits and other issues in their lives. It also suggests that the more challenges young people face, the more time they need to address those issues. The notions of reparatory responsibility and foundational rights justify extending support beyond attainment of legal adulthood where young people are unable to overcome the challenges they face during the period of their childhood. In the following discussion, I first address the tendency for recent policy initiatives to prioritise or reward 'successful' young people rather than targeting the highest levels of support to those for whom the conditions required for 'full' autonomy remain out of reach. I argue for a more individual response to young people's needs and consider the barriers to such an approach imposed by the nature of 'corporate parenting'.

Corporate parenting and the '"deserving"– "undeserving" schism'

To an extent, the apparent shift of emphasis in English policy in favour of more successful young people reflects the progress that has been made in encouraging high aspirations and in supporting care leavers to fulfil their potential. It is indicative of the relative success of the initiatives of the last 15 to 20 years and, as such, is cause for celebration. Mr Brook reported a change in focus from young people at risk of becoming NEET to considera-tion of the need to do more to ensure sure that 'more able' students fulfilled their potential at 'A' level and in higher education, driven by the increas-ing proportion of children in care in Riversmeet achieving well at GCSE. Ms Ford was 'targeting' children in Wadebridge who had been identified 'as going on to higher education'. Mr Steel recounted taking an individual interest in a young man who appeared to be capable of university entry and described the additional work needed now that more young people were do-ing well enough to be able to pick and choose post-16 courses. This attention by virtual head-teachers in part arose from the fact that social workers and carers may have very little experience of supporting young people aiming at higher education. However, while these scenarios in themselves indicate significant progress for some young people in care, they do not justify less attention and resources being invested in the most disadvantaged.

The accordance of privilege to more successful young people was not gen-erally reflected in interviews with participating professionals, but it is rather apparent from the wider policy context, from the experiences of young peo-ple excluded from mainstream school and/or college, and from accounts of some financially driven decisions around placement moves. Three possible drivers come to mind, all of which may be influential. The first lies in the imposition of greater managerialism and regulation associated with neo-liberal principles. These have led to the 'outcome-driven' policies which impose targets and measure success in concrete terms such as the number of GCSEs children attain at grades A*-C. Under such regimes, institutions are perversely led to focus on children at the margins of measurable suc-cess, removing attention and resources from those for whom the selected measure is unattainable (Gillborn and Youdell, 2000). From an institutional perspective, it is not 'worth' investing in those students, because there is little likelihood of a successful 'return' on that investment for the institution (the school or corporate parent). While local authorities have been judged by the proportion of care leavers who are NEET at 19 for some time, this is not a target that impacts directly on schools, which are incentivized not to keep low-achieving or poorly behaved students on roll, and there is now data collected on the number of care leavers progressing to higher educa-tion. Such schemes tend only to be sensitive to population-level measures, overlooking the needs and characteristics of individuals and exemplifying the reproduction of power or disadvantage by state institutions (Fineman, 2008). These ideas are also associated with marketization principles such as incentivisation, as discussed in Chapter 2 in relation to schemes in England, the US and Hungary which provide or provided preferential services to care leavers continuing in education or training, thereby perversely discriminat-ing against those young people who are ineligible by reason of their limited educational attainment for access to those services, although by definition they are most in need of support (House of Commons Children, Schools and Families Committee, 2009).

The second possibility has its roots in what appears to be a peculiarly Anglophone tendency (Fionda, 2005) to demonise certain subsections of the youth population. Much has been written about the highly artificial distinction between children who are 'troubled' (the domain of social care services, and including children in the care system) and children who are 'troublesome', particularly children in trouble with the law (Goldson and Muncie, 2006). Broadhurst et al. (2009), among others, point to the way in which New Labour's linkage of rights with responsibilities justified a punitive response to those children and young people – often the most marginalized – exhibiting problematic behaviour. Children from a care background are more likely than their peers in the general population to have been exposed to the risk factors associated with youth offending, including lack of parental support and poor school attendance, and they are disproportionately represented in the criminal justice system internationally (Kennedy, 2013; Berlin et al., 2011; Cutuli et al., 2016). In this study, at least four of the young men had been involved with the police and/or implicated in incidents of violence (Callum, Luis, Niall and Riley). Goldson (2000: 262) described the punitive stance of youth justice policy introduced under New Labour as 'fundamentally antipathetic to the principles of the Children Act 1989' and warned of the risk that it would lead to 'the abrogation of professional responsibilities towards "children in need"', a group he defines broadly, to include care leavers. Thus, there may be an inherent propensity in professional practice towards Goldson's '"deserving"–"undeserving" schism', in which young people regarded as 'troublesome' are deemed unworthy of state support. Analysis using the concepts of reparatory responsibility and foundational rights exposes the falseness, not to say hypocrisy, of such distinctions. Rather than holding such young people to account for their actions at an early age, the concept of foundational rights suggests that the most vulnerable young people should carry less (legal) responsibility for their behaviour, because they are furthest from achieving the conditions needed to exercise 'full' autonomy.

In a consumerist education sector, in which schools compete through league tables of assessment criteria, it would be unsurprising if schools were not acutely aware of the distinction between 'good' pupils and 'troublesome' pupils. In the CLET study, it was clear from interviews with designated teachers that children in care were generally regarded as 'troublesome' and expected to exhibit challenging behaviour. The way in which designated teachers explained their role demonstrated their understanding of the implications of this tendency and also that they readily accepted responsibility for encouraging their colleagues to be more understanding of the background circumstances of these children. Designated teachers described the need to 'explain our children to the teachers', as Mr Brown put it, and they spent considerable time and energy advocating against their exclusion.

Those participants that remained in mainstream schools or colleges unquestionably had better prospects than those that did not at the end of the study: all nine of those categorised as 'Moving On' remained in mainstream education throughout the study. Of course it is impossible to demonstrate that mainstream education is primarily responsible for the more promising outlooks for this group, as those excluded from mainstream settings will have been more 'troublesome' (and therefore troubled) on the whole than those who were not. However, excluding Ollie, who was in a special school as a result of his significant disabilities, seven of the 20 young people were excluded from school or college (Gilroy, Habib, Luis, Niall, Qadira, Riley and Unity), in addition to Farouk having been excluded from a private college due to his immigration status. These findings reflect an international trend of children in state care being at greater risk of exclusion than their peers (O'Higgins et al., 2015). They are of particular concern in the English context because statutory guidance on the role of the designated teacher for local authorities published after the conclusion of the CLET study (DfE, 2014: 13) appears weaker than the earlier version (DCSF, 2009), advising merely that 'headteachers should, as far as possible, avoid excluding any looked-after child'.

Once children were excluded, designated teachers in non-mainstream settings described a tendency for schools to abdicate responsibility for those children to the alternative setting: Ms Tan went so far as to describe the children she worked with as having been 'put in the bin of life'. Exclusion from school is almost certain to cause considerable disruption in a young person's life, particularly in their peer relationships, but also potentially affects their care placement. The focal model reminds us that imposing such additional challenging life changes on vulnerable young people at critical moments in their educational trajectory is likely to be more than they can successfully negotiate, potentially triggering a downward spiral of challenging behaviour and poor focus on schoolwork described by professional participants. In this study, my strong impression from three interviews with Callum was that, without the extremely understanding response of the school to his acutely challenging behaviour, Callum's prospects would have been extremely poor.

The third possible driver for the tendency to prioritise 'good' young people over those regarded as 'troublesome' relates to the concept of 'agency neglect', a term coined in recent years to describe the reluctance of professionals to engage with the most difficult adolescents (Brandon et al., 2008). Such young people are especially challenging to work with or 'hard to help' and require specialist carers and intensive intervention. Engagement in education is not realistic until their lives have been 'sorted out' as Priya put it, or, to use the words of Ms Mason, 'there are all kinds of things that need to go in first before there's going to be any kind of fruitful learning or engagement'. Once again these accounts align with the focal model of adolescence, although in many cases young people may need therapeutic intervention in order to move on from trauma. These young people have typically experienced a history of loss and rejection coupled with long-term maltreatment (Brandon et al., 2008). Attention to the life circumstances of this very vulnerable group exposes the false dichotomy of the 'troubled' or 'troublesome' child and of the '"deserving"–"undeserving" schism'. In the context of care leavers, the concept of 'agency neglect' draws attention to the deficiencies in the exercise of the parental responsibility that the state holds for this unique group. It also highlights the particular importance of the relational aspects of autonomy developed by Nussbaum (2003) and Hollingsworth (2013b). The application of foundational rights theory in the context of the focal model of adolescence suggests that the state's duties to care leavers are heaviest towards those in greatest need of reparation for the state's failure to protect them from parental maltreatment or inadequacies. The next section considers in greater detail how the local authority corporate parent should enact those duties and the challenges in doing so effectively in both social care and education.

Corporate parenting and individual children

Bullock et al. (2006: 1349) conclude that 'the "state" as an impersonal entity clearly cannot provide the day-to-day care that would normally be taken to constitute "parenting"' (see also Bluff et al., 2012). They also point out that the factors predicting success in long-term care placements are similar to those applicable to birth parent families but that successful outcomes are particularly difficult to achieve for children in long-term foster placements and older children who are likely to be viewed as 'troublesome'. Focusing on relational interpretations of capabilities and/or the relational aspects of autonomy reinforces the importance to the child of the corporate parent having a human face (see, for example, the experiences of care leavers at university reported in Jackson et al., 2005). For the vast majority of children, parental responsibility vests in at least one and probably two adults, usually the child's birth parents. The adult who makes day-to-day decisions with or on behalf of the child is also the person who cares most for and about them and with whom they have the closest relationship. In the case of children in care, parental responsibility vests in the elected members and council officers of the local authority. Most local authorities now have a corporate parenting board or group and some have established 'multi-agency looked after partnerships' (Hart and Williams, 2013). However, Ofsted (2011: 148) concluded that '[t]oo many local authorities...lacked a robust strategy for corporate parenting' and that corporate parenting boards in some areas were still in the early stages of development. Ofsted (2013a) has also expressed concern that nearly a third of local authorities had experienced one or more changes in the identity of the director of children's services in the course of a year. In the CLET study, the virtual head of Stonycross, Ms Mason, reported a 'massive changeover of senior managers', so that all the people who had set up the virtual school had left.

The number of children for whom an English corporate parent is responsible varies widely from none in the Isles of Scilly to well over a thousand in Birmingham (DfE/NS, 2016a), giving some corporate parents responsibility for an exceptionally large and diverse 'family'. Ofsted (2013a: 6) concluded that 'overall trends of improvement mask failings for individual children'. The question therefore, is whether, and if so how, the corporate parenting model, however manifested in different national contexts, can provide children with individually sensitive and responsive exercise of parental responsibility and with a consistent and caring relationship with a supportive adult, or whether, in reality, effective parental responsibility can only be exercised by an individual adult with a close and caring relationship with the child.

At the least, it is imperative that young people are provided with a social care professional who has the time and skills to be able to develop a meaningful relationship with the young person and is a consistent figure in their lives over time. This has been the Achilles heel of the English care system for too long. Following the Munro review (2011), attention has been paid to strengthening social work training, including through specific incorporation of the skills and capabilities required for child and family social work into professional training (Department for Education, 2011). Munro also exhorted a return to relationship-based practice in social work, which had reputedly become more and more desk-bound with the introduction of case management processes. However, the child and family social work profession remains afflicted by a long-term shortage in supply, high turnover and short professional life, low morale, perceived high case-loads, excessive paperwork and limited opportunities for promotion at the frontline (Holmes et al., 2013).

In the early help assessment model adopted after the Munro review and incorporated in *Working Together*, the multi-agency statutory guidance for child protection (HM Government, 2015), a lead professional is appointed to manage co-ordinated assessment and support for families, and a similar model governs the development and delivery of child protection plans. Both of these processes are likely to be relatively short-term interventions, and the child usually remains at home with their family throughout. The challenges in relation to assuring consistency and personal attention to the needs of children in care throughout their childhood are significantly greater, but there have been a number of policy initiatives in recent years to attempt to address them, including the introduction of Independent Reviewing Officers and the recent devolution of decision-making to carers.

Independent Reviewing Officers (IROs) were introduced by the Adoption and Children Act 2002 s118 to chair review meetings in order to ensure that care plans were effectively implemented. They were given power to refer cases in which the care plan had not been adequately followed to the Child and Family Court Advisory and Support Service (Cafcass) with a view to an appropriate application being made to the court, for example for discharge of the care order. This scheme appeared however to be ineffective (Fortin, 2009), and the responsibilities of Independent Reviewing Officers to monitor the implementation of care plans were strengthened through the Children and Young Persons Act 2008 and the Care Planning, Placement and Case Review (England) Regulations 2010. Although IROs are now required to monitor the general performance of the corporate parent and alert senior managers to inadequate practice in the care of children and management of case planning, the role remains that of an officer of the local authority, and in its response to the Family Justice Review Interim Report (Family Justice Review Panel, 2011), the National Association of Independent Reviewing Officers (NAIRO) expressed concern that some IROs report being 'encouraged to tone down or suppress concerns they have about local authority plans and practice' (Fayle, 2011: 4). Ofsted, too, have concluded that the role is underdeveloped and that IROs need to be supported to challenge corporate parenting in order to drive improvement in practice (Ofsted, 2013b).

Research by the National Children's Bureau (Jelicic et al., 2014) in four local authority areas has found variable performance. The findings highlight the importance of IROs building meaningful relationships with children in order to advocate for them, but some children felt that there was no point in informing their IRO of their wishes and feelings as they would not be acted upon. The recommendations of young people contributing to the research make salutary reading and include: 'IROs should not judge CYP [children and young people] and they should leave any personal feelings out of the situation. Care leavers are *not* typical young people and require more understanding and patience from professionals' (97). Many young people appear only to have contact with their IRO at the time of their six-monthly reviews (Jelicic et al., 2014). In the CLET study, young people rarely mentioned their IROs, and none appeared to regard them as of particular significance. The IRO role may, therefore, have as yet unrealised potential to improve corporate parenting practice but does not currently appear to be a realistic means through which both of the dual aspects of parenting – which might loosely be categorised as responsibility and care – might be embodied.

Since this study, regulations have been amended to require the delegation of day-to-day decisions to foster carers or residential care workers (taking into account the child's views and respecting their own decision-making capacity) and to ensure that carers are treated in the same way as birth parents for the purposes of information-sharing and consent to participation in school activities. These changes may alleviate some of the frustrations surrounding delayed approval of plans described by young people in this study and perhaps enhance children's sense of family belonging. However, in themselves they cannot address the strategic failings in corporate parenting that currently lead to poor placements, multiple moves or placements far from the child's home area, nor will they materially assist young people who do not have a good relationship with their foster carer. Further, where parental responsibility and care are separated, children and carers are likely to continue to be subjected to the intrusive surveillance described by participants in this study, such as Tasmin, and it is less likely that decisions will be taken with a full understanding of an individual child's wishes and feelings.

Where young people have strong and enduring relationships with their foster carers, such as that enjoyed by Jacinda, perhaps greater consideration could be given to the use of Special Guardianship Orders, which take children out of state care, although they may continue to be eligible for leaving care services if the order is made when they are over 16 but under 21 (Children Act 1989, s24). Under s14, local authority foster carers can apply for a Special Guardianship Order in relation to a child who has lived with them for at least a year preceding the application. The special guardian obtains parental responsibility through the order, which they may exercise to the exclusion of that of others, but (contrary to the English position in relation to adoption) the birth parents do not lose parental responsibility. In the CLET study, Devora's carer obtained a Special Guardianship Order, but she was Devora's cousin. Research has found little use of this provision by stranger foster carers, probably due to concerns about financial and social services support to special guardians (Wade et al., 2014). However the research predates case law which made clear that local authorities must have regard to the fostering allowance, which would have been payable if the child were fostered, in assessing the support paid to special guardians (*R (on the application of TT) v London Borough of Merton* [2012]). Most recently, children leaving care for a private law order such as Special Guardianship or into adoption will be come under the virtual school for the purposes of promotion of their educational achievement (Children Act 1989, s23ZZA as amended by the Children and Social Work Act 2017).

The Children and Young People (Scotland) Act 2014 s19 attempted to introduce a 'named person service', in which an identified individual employed by the local authority (such as a teacher) is to be available to all children of school age to advise, inform and support the child or their parent (employees of the health service such as health visitors would provide a similar service for pre-school children). Implementation of the scheme was stalled by the Supreme Court on the basis of an objection that the information-sharing provisions rendered it in breach of article 8 of the European Convention on Human Rights (rights to privacy and family life) (*The Christian Institute and others v The Lord Advocate (Scotland)* [2016]), but the Scottish government was seeking to roll the service out in 2018 at the time of writing (Deputy First Minister, 2017). Although the difficulties inherent in the designated teacher role have been explored in this book, the named person role is a wider one in terms of advice and support extending across all areas of a child's life. Where all children are given access to a named professional in this way, there should be less stigma for children in care in taking advantage of the role, which could be more intensive in relation to more vulnerable groups of children.

Alternatively, social workers could be appointed to schools to fulfil a similar named person role, which would bring a number of advantages. First, social workers within schools would provide a bridge between social care and education services within the local authority and enhance multi-agency working with respect to child protection and safeguarding concerns and referrals as well as for children in state care. Second, embedding social work as a more generic service would help to lift the stigma associated with receipt of social care services which has blighted safeguarding work in this country for so many years. Third, if the social worker allocated to their case was based in a child's school, he or she would be more readily available and have greater opportunities to interact outside statutory review requirements, which tended to be experienced by young people in this study as serving the needs of the corporate parent rather than the child. Social worker roles embedded in schools would be likely to be more stable than those within local authority children's social care teams in the current environment. Social workers were employed in a few schools in this study, but the trend appeared to be withdrawal of the service at a time of budget cuts. There are similar arrangements in some other jurisdictions, such as the Child and Family Support Team Initiative in North Carolina, in which school-based nurses and social workers jointly support children at risk of school failure or out-of-home care (Gifford et al., 2010). In the US, attempts to fund such initiatives through a proposed School Social Workers Improving Student Success Act (H.R. 563 113th Congress and H.R. 2988 114th Congress) were unsuccessful. Another possible model would be based on existing systems to support migrant children, such as the Scottish independent guardian model for UASC introduced by the Human Trafficking and Exploitation (Scotland) Act 2015, or the independent child trafficking advocate model under the Modern Slavery Act 2015 in England, which is available for children who have been or are suspected to have been trafficked or identified as at risk of trafficking. Scottish guardians help young people negotiate all aspects of their new lives, including legal advice for asylum application, accommodation and education and liaise with services on their behalf (Edinburgh Peace and Justice Centre, 2016).

Corporate parenting and education

The diversity of experiences and needs amongst care leavers makes it difficult to make generalisations about the effect of education policy on the cohort as a whole. Further, in the educational arena, the English corporate parent may have potentially conflicting responsibilities to the children in its education system who are not in care and those for whom it has direct parental responsibility. The numbers of children in care in many individual schools are low, making this group less likely to be a priority for head-teachers. Consistent with the argument above that young people are unique individuals requiring the personal guidance and care of adults who know and understand them, this section focuses on the extent to which recent policy developments enable professionals and the education estate to understand

and respond sensitively to young people's particular circumstances in order to support their education and promote their educational attainment.

The role of the designated teacher

The elevation of the role of the designated teacher to a statutory footing has guaranteed a single point of responsibility for this cohort at a senior level within each school. The designated teachers in mainstream schools in the CLET study played a key role in managing the tensions arising from young people's pastoral needs spilling over into the school environment in a climate of pressure on schools to maintain high standards of attainment and behaviour. It appears that ensuring the role is held at a senior level within the school may allow the holder to be an effective advocate for those young people who do not always find it easy to conform to behavioural expectations or focus on their studies. Many examples of effective intervention within school by designated teachers were apparent, the most striking being in relation to 'fighting' for young people not to be excluded. The study also found evidence of the value of the role in managing information-sharing within and beyond the school and in petitioning social care services on behalf of children, for example where disruptive placement moves were planned, either directly or through the local authority virtual head. The external-facing aspect of the designated teacher role may be particularly important where social work staff are transient and/or have limited contact with young people.

However, the high number of young people participating in the study who had been excluded from school or college suggests that professional participants in the study may have been unusually motivated and confident in advocating on behalf of children. This tentative finding is reinforced by Mr Brook's comment that some designated teachers are 'struggling to find their voice in schools' and Mr Steel's acknowledgment of high numbers of children in the care of Ironbridge in Pupil Referral Units. The seniority of designated teachers within the school hierarchy was seen as important by designated teachers and virtual heads to ensure that the needs of young people are addressed both individually and strategically. Calvert (2009) describes the development of pastoral care within schools from a position of low status to one in which it has been explicitly linked to learning and in which non-teachers undertake roles that are central to child well-being. The designated teacher post appears to fit neatly into this trajectory in the prioritisation of educational attainment in the functions of the role. However, teachers who are ambitious for their own career progression may find it difficult to reconcile their commitment to meeting the school's performance management targets with their responsibility to protect the broader best interests of children in care.

Other potential disadvantages of the designated teacher post being held at a high level of seniority in the school are evident from the study. The professional identity of teachers and the hierarchical structure of schools is very different from the ethos of social care, and the more senior the teacher, the more difficult and perhaps inappropriate it may be for a teacher to be involved directly in pastoral care. In some cases, young people's aspirations and plans were not known to designated teachers, who had made assumptions about their appropriate career trajectories based on their academic potential rather than their personal interests. Young people were extremely reluctant to be treated differently from their peers in any respect and could feel oppressively monitored or singled out, reflecting Power's observation (1996) that pastoral care mechanisms in school may become a vehicle for control and surveillance.

For the most part, therefore, young people had little to do with their designated teachers, beyond fulfilling what they saw as largely administrative requirements imposed by Personal Education Plan review meetings. The exception to this model in mainstream schools was Mr Brown, who was semi-retired and held a non-teaching role. He was clearly someone in whom young people were readily able to confide. In general, therefore, this study supports the suggestion of Fletcher-Campbell (2008) that the different aspects of the designated teacher role might best be undertaken by more than one member of the school staff. It is also possible that the tensions recounted above might be less acute in an educational environment less preoccupied with attainment outcomes, where all children are accepted as members of the school community and schools are under less pressure to remove poorly performing or disruptive children from their roll. Ms Gold's expressed discomfort with the emphasis of the statutory guidance on promoting high expectations on the basis that 'it should be the same for everyone' is founded on a concern that the ethos of schools should ensure that *all* children are equally valued and supported in order to achieve in line with their personal potential. It is apparent that the school environment has enormous potential to provide support through the consistent rhythm of school life and the young person's sense of 'attachment' to the school community (if established), but relationships with teachers cannot be expected to compensate for deficiencies in those with social workers or carers. In all the study schools, much investment had been made to increase the pastoral support to such young people through social workers, pastoral leaders or mentors, but these models were under threat from budgetary pressures.

A weakness of the designated teacher role apparent from this study was the limited extent to which schools were directly involved in young people's transition to college at 16, which was regarded as the preserve of the leaving care team and was also hampered by poor or non-existent relationships between schools and further education colleges. This is an area which might be significantly strengthened by: focused oversight by virtual heads (discussed below); development of arrangements for care leavers at further education colleges; and adoption of some of the strategies used by head-teachers in non-mainstream settings in this study.

In the non-mainstream settings, which were for the most part very small, responsibility for children in care (who often comprised a high proportion of the school's population) lay with the head-teacher. All five participants working in non-mainstream settings therefore had considerable expertise in responding to the needs of children in care but tended not to see them as a discrete group because all members of the school had unique needs. In some ways this was an advantage in that all children were regarded as individuals and none felt singled out within that environment. However, with the exception of Ms Coral, there was little engagement with the local virtual school, seemingly for a variety of reasons, including that the school was independent or because engagement with social services was primarily through the Special Educational Needs service. Establishing robust links between virtual schools and designated or named teachers in alternative provision should be a first step to ensuring that individual attention is given to planning the educational progression of young people out of mainstream school. On the evidence from Forest Hill College, similar arrangements with senior members of staff at further education colleges have the potential to improve retention rates at college.

The introduction of virtual school head-teachers

The CLET study was conducted at a time when the population of children in care in England was rising rapidly (DfE/NS, 2011), yet local authorities were suffering from ongoing austerity measures which disproportionately affected children's social care, especially in authorities with high numbers of children in care (Chartered Institute of Public Finance and Accountancy, 2011). In agreement with the findings of Ofsted (2012) in relation to inspections of nine local authorities, professional participants in the CLET study reported significant budget cuts. One participating virtual school had lost its dedicated 16-plus transitions officer in budget cuts and funding for a project to reduce the number of care leavers who are NEET had run out in another; in a third, the resources and staffing budget for children in care had been cut by 50–60 per cent. While introduction of a statutory requirement for local authorities to appoint a virtual school head (or analogous post) (Children Act 1989 s22(3B)) to monitor the fulfilment of the local authority's duty to promote the educational achievement of children in care is extremely welcome, it should be noted that a single appointment is sufficient to meet the statutory requirement. It was evident from the CLET study that the participating local authorities were extremely stretched. All virtual heads were part-time in that role (see Table 1.4 in Appendix 1) and most had other responsibilities, as well as very small teams. Ms Coral said of her local authority virtual school:

> The virtual team were excellent...but they were horrifically under-staffed, and at one point it was just the head of the virtual school who was functioning on her own, with one temporary agency member of

staff...with some of the children who were seriously at risk she would attend the meetings herself, but she was stretched incredibly thin.

Nonetheless, implementation of this role on a statutory basis recognises the importance of education in improving the prospects of children in care. On the evidence of the CLET study, virtual school heads are well-placed to co-ordinate work and ensure effective communication between education and social care, particularly in relation to attendance and the avoidance of exclusion – endorsing the conclusions of Ofsted (2011, 2012) – and in relation to transition planning.

Virtual heads in this study acknowledged that this group of children is un-likely to be a priority for head-teachers in mainstream schools. Overall, they felt that significant progress had been made since the virtual school system was instituted in the sensitivity with which schools responded to the needs of children in care. Despite the variety of structures in different local au-thorities, a number of strengths common to all the models can be identified. All teams were multi-disciplinary or embedded within a multi-disciplinary structure: in Wadebridge for example, that included an education psycholo-gist as well as members from the SEN team, educational welfare and social care and a head-teacher, in order to link up practice across the authority. Virtual schools modelled themselves on school leadership teams, and par-ticipants stressed that they also deliberately mirrored schools in the way in which children were monitored: 'we now feel that we are a school, and we are tracking our pupils, etc., etc. in the same way that a school would do' (Ms Mason). All prioritised monitoring of attendance to ensure that they were informed immediately if children were not in school and collected at-tainment data on 'their' children regularly. Ms Mason considered that this enabled the virtual school to be much more proactive, rather than primarily responding to crises brought to them by social workers. The focus was re-lentlessly on attainment: 'the priority is always trying to raise achievement of young people, that's...how we are measured, both by central, and locally' (Mr Brook); 'the emphasis is about attainment, and outcomes, quite frankly, about what they are going to do when they come out of school' (Ms Lea).

Another common aspect of their role concerned empowering social work-ers to challenge schools. Virtual heads paid particular attention to ensuring that social workers and foster carers are equipped to act as would educated, knowledgeable parents, including in understanding the system of attain-ment levels, the complex qualifications available at 16 and over and working with further education colleges. Ms Ford described some of the social work-ers as feeling 'quite intimidated' by schools, which they felt 'weren't being as cooperative as they could be'. She said 'social workers don't have that confidence...they won't challenge a head teacher'. Social workers and teach-ers 'don't speak the same language necessarily' (Ms Mason), but as former senior teachers, members of the virtual schools were comfortable commu-nicating in schools and found schools were much more willing to engage with them than with social workers. Ms Ford felt her team had succeeded in 'raising the profile' of children in care within schools and enabling social workers to challenge schools. She also commented that teachers seemed to prefer to approach her with questions rather than social workers.

Current priorities varied amongst the virtual heads, but a common issue raised by virtual schools was that of enabling children to make smooth educational transitions when moving care placements. This was a particular issue where children were placed out of the local authority area, an issue also identified by Ofsted (2012). The care of children placed outside their 'home' local authority has been an issue of concern in its own right for some years. Ofsted (2014) has highlighted deficiencies in the quality of care, information-sharing, direct support for a child's particular needs and contact with their birth family for this group of children. Ms Ford estimated that just over half of 'her' secondary children were in placement out-of-area, requiring her to travel 'all the way around the country' to meet them. In part, that was because the authority was small and unable to find placements in the local authority area for all children, but in some cases it was a deliberate decision to place the child at some distance from their birth family. Additionally, there were no residential homes in her authority, so eight secondary-age children were out-of-area in specialist schools to meet their particular needs. Although she felt they were getting an 'excellent education', such arrangements can introduce further complications. Ms Mason commented:

> particularly with statemented pupils...not only are you working with another local authority, but you often have to go through your own SEN department, their SEN department, two lots of complex needs panels... it's a bit of a minefield.

Developing post-16 provision was an area of focus for virtual heads: it is now imperative that all virtual schools extend at least to 18, and preferably to 25, to match the corporate parent's obligations under the Children and Young Persons Act 2008 and the Children and Social Work Act 2017. A common issue at Stonycross, where about 35 per cent of children in the virtual school had SEN statements, was a failure for support to be continued post-16 through a Learning Difficulties Assessment:

> a lot of them, when they leave school at Year 11, don't have a Section 139 assessment, so you might get statements finishing but no further support gets identified, and of course that leads to all sorts of problems when they go on to vocational training or college courses... If they were ours we'd be making sure that those all happened, you know.

Although stressing that they operated like a school, virtual heads spoke about the children in their school from a parental perspective. Ms Mason, for example, commented on the complexities of placing children out of area, saying: 'because we are the parent, we would like our children to be dealt with in a particular way, but there's no way through that sometimes'. All virtual heads appeared to take a very personal interest in 'their' children, including attending personal education plan meetings where appropriate, organising achievement or celebration days and offering personal guidance to young people considering application to university. Ms Ford at Wadebridge had taken over all Personal Education Plan (PEP) meetings in order to get to know the children personally, raise the profile of the virtual school within schools and ensure appropriate support was in place. She did not think that would be sustainable in the long-term, but in the short-term it enabled her to make relationships with schools and children and challenge schools directly. She also planned to accompany students to university interviews if it was needed, although commented that often the foster carers were very good at doing that.

The virtual school system therefore appears to offer some opportunity for the local authority to present a human face to children in care and to provide some of the personal care and individual attention that young people need. Wadebridge was implementing a 'Care to Work' plan, taking a holistic approach to all aspects of a young person's life and incorporating the 'Grow our Own' group offering work experience and skills development within the authority itself, demonstrating the potential for local authorities to take a more 'hands on' approach to corporate parenting. The 'pupil premium', additional funding to support vulnerable groups, is now paid directly to virtual schools, and Ms Ford took care to account for the individual needs of each child, such as providing horse-riding for a young woman over the summer holidays before she started at equine college to ensure that her riding skills were adequate.

Although virtual schools' rolls include all children in schools or colleges in the local area, at the time of the study, increasing numbers of schools were becoming academies, which are funded by central government rather than the local authority. Professional participants were concerned as to the effect of such independently operating schools on a range of issues, including ensuring that children in care are provided with the right school placement in a timely fashion, managing attendance, preventing exclusion where at all possible, arranging for young people who are not able to function successfully in a mainstream school to be given the highest quality alternative placement and prepared for return to mainstream education at the earliest opportunity and ensuring that excluded young people are not overlooked but that their educational progression is planned and supported as it would be for any other young person. There was speculation that academies might in future be required to pay for the services of the virtual school, which is part of the local authority. Ms Mason's view was that 'the idea that any schools are going to commission our services is ludicrous...because half the time they haven't got any looked-after children, and...as a head, I know that it wouldn't be, probably, top of my list'. This model may not therefore translate directly into other systems in which local area education and social care systems are separate, without careful attention to the structural arrangements.

A holistic approach: the social pedagogy model

All the roles discussed above focus on either the child's care *or* their education, and the introduction of more individuals with specific, specialised responsibilities – such as the designated teacher and the IRO – into a child's life may operate to reinforce feelings of self-reliance because of the inevitable sense of intrusion, dilution of relationships and accompanying administrative tasks. The literature from a number of perspectives including attachment and resilience theory is clear that children in care need a strong caring relationship with at least one consistent adult in their lives. This may be attainable through the traditional Anglophone social worker model, but only with significant investment to provide intensive, relationship-based practice and a stable workforce (McLeod, 2010). Recent interest in social pedagogy in the UK appears to have sprung from concerns around the separation of the care, education, health and justice sectors; the professional skills and morale of the children's social care workforce; and inadequate attention to adult–child relationships in social work (Coussée et al., 2010). Yet, despite the fact that the cross-disciplinary and cross-agency nature of social pedagogy practice makes it well-suited to contribute to the development of policy and practice in children's social care work, the movement in the UK has relied largely on grass-roots projects with little interest from government beyond a pilot scheme in residential care in 2008 (Petrie, 2013).

The professional remit of social pedagogy comprises a number of distinguishing characteristics that are arguably deficient in English practice, including attention to the child's emerging citizenship and their relationship with society, the use of physical care and comfort and the combined use of intellectual and practical skills with compassionate practice ('heart, head, hands') (Cameron, 2004). Kemp argues that social pedagogy 'provides a *coherent ethical* framework for policy, and professional education and practice' and in particular acknowledges the central role of relationships of trust and of empathy in social care practice (Kemp, 2015: 348). While these are strengths which would potentially benefit practice in the UK and other English-speaking contexts, critics point out that the individualistic approach to children's well-being in these nations is incompatible with the focus on the social world of the social pedagogic approach and would be liable to undermine attempts to draw on it (Smith and Whyte, 2008; Coussée et al., 2010) without specific attention to development of theory and practice that is context-specific (Petrie, 2013). Coussée et al. (2010) argue that the concept of 'corporate parenting' in principle has potential to promote the social-pedagogic notion of children's upbringing as a shared societal responsibility, but only if there is a shift from expectations that individuals' problems and behaviour can be managed by expert intervention to a broader understanding of the implications of the social context. In Scotland, Smith and Whyte (2008) consider that a more socioeducational conceptualisation of social problems, which attends to the broader social context, and a less distinct separation of disciplines of care and education render the context more amenable to development of a social pedagogical approach than is the case in England.

Boddy (2011), however, argues that social pedagogy is particularly well-suited to relational work with children in care for a number of reasons: first, because attachment work with maltreated children requires more than ordinary 'good' parenting; second, because of the particular importance of building sustained relationships in carefully matched and stable placements; third, because some children, including older children and large siblings groups, may not be suited to, or able to find a placement in, foster care; and fourth, because many placements in the English context are task-focused rather than concerned with the long-term upbringing of children. Further, the social pedagogic model explicitly addresses the tension between the personal and professional aspects of caring for children of the state (Boddy, 2011), providing children with carers who combine the necessary professional expertise and a reflective capacity with personal empathy and practical engagement. While there has been some development in English-speaking contexts of more professional foster placements, such as Treatment Foster Care Oregon (see e.g. Sinclair et al., 2016), these are often task-focused in that they may be introduced to address specific behavioural difficulties, for example. The social pedagogue's relationship with children is not only concerned with their upbringing and education in the broadest sense but is also founded on participatory principles of dialogue and equality to promote emotional development, self-reflection and engagement with the wider society. These aspects of the social pedagogic approach resonate with Nussbaum's definitions of the central human capabilities of 'Emotions' and 'Affiliation', suggesting that the social pedagogic approach is better-suited to pay attention to the relational aspects of autonomy and foundational rights than Anglophone models.

Conclusion

Ms Oak said of some of the young people she was aware of at Forest Hill College, who still came within the remit of the virtual school at 20 or 21, that 'they are adults, obviously, legally, but they are still young people who haven't got the skills for life yet'. There is much to praise in recent initiatives within education that have focused individual attention on young people's educational progress and attainment. Arguably the virtual head role provides a powerful contribution to corporate parenting in this regard. However, two interrelated concerns stand out: the first is that, given the interdependence of the two, there is a risk that progress made in recent years in relation to education for children in care may be undermined by less effective social care practice. I will return to this point after addressing the second, which relates to those young people who, at a time when academic attainment for the cohort as a whole appears to be improving, remain in the margins of educational provision and social inclusion. Although it should be noted that three of the girls participating in the study were accessed through a specialist provider of services for care leavers requiring a high level of support, it is concerning that nine of the 21 young participants were excluded from and/or dropped out of, school and/or college. Using Hollingsworth's terminology, this constitutes a failure in the state's exercise of its assumed responsibility for the children entrusted to its care.

Overall, this study paints a picture of some care leavers doing very well educationally and appearing to be well-equipped for adulthood, while others, who may be hard to help or find themselves on the wrong side of the '"deserving"–"undeserving" schism', still face a very bleak future. The period covered by this study, particularly for those leaving school at 16, is likely to be crucial in shaping their future prospects. It is clear that there is much more that could be done by local authorities and further education colleges in exercise of the state's reparatory responsibility to support vulnerable young people through this transition and beyond, in fulfilment of young people's foundational rights. Since the study was conducted, there has been some erosion of policies according preferential treatment to more educationally successful young people. At the time of the CLET study, national policy explicitly entitled young people aged 21–24 and continuing in education or training to greater support than their peers. While the specific requirements on the local authority to support care leavers' education and training remain, the Children and Social Work Act 2017 has levelled the playing field in terms of identical entitlements for all 21–24 year-olds to a pathway plan, personal advisor and assessment. This change in legislative duties reflects a recognition in national policy of the need to support extended pathways to independence, not just for young people whose transition to independence is prolonged by further and higher education, but for all care leavers.

It is to be hoped that it also reflects a move away from the '"deserving"–"undeserving" schism', although this appears to be entrenched in many aspects of policy in neoliberal nations. The significance of situating children's experiences within the social context in social pedagogic work is critical to the avoidance of a culture of individual responsibility and blame that the '"deserving"–"undeserving" schism' exemplifies, and Coussée et al. (2010: 100) caution that without attention to that aspect of social pedagogy, relationship-based and empathetic practice risk becoming no more than 'useful "tools" for fitting delinquent or disturbed children and young people to educational or economical priorities'. But there are other challenges to introducing social pedagogic principles into practice in English-speaking contexts. In English-speaking countries outside the UK, there is very limited knowledge of social pedagogy (Moss and Cameron, 2011), but neoliberal models of working which are hierarchical and driven by principles of marketization such as efficiency, commodification and outcome-measurement are antithetical to a profession in which individual situational judgement is trusted and the child is an equal partner in a collaborative endeavour. Moss and Cameron conclude that the low status of 'care work' in those nations renders the task of moving to a higher-status, professional workforce challenging not only by reason of cost but also because of the change in values and attitudes required, including in relation to the value accorded to the work and the need to shift from increasing role specialization to a holistic and relationship-based approach, in which physical care is not demeaning but an integral part of bringing up children. However, the social pedagogic approach has considerable potential to reconcile the tensions between corporate responsibility and individual care in its combination of professional expertise with personal relationships and its focus beyond individual responsibility for measured outcomes to a broader understanding of young people's social contexts and attention to social justice. In the final chapter, I consider further the implications of the findings of the CLET study for international practice in the education and care of children ageing out of care and suggest ways forward for research and practice.

9   Conclusion

Introduction

Internationally, research into care leavers' needs, experiences and outcomes in early adulthood remains patchy, and it is unclear to what extent care improves the life chances of its graduates (Maclean et al., 2016). In their systematic review of literature comparing outcomes for out-of-home care with in-home care for maltreated children, Maclean et al. highlight issues of selection bias inherent in research in this area, since children in out-of-home care should by definition be at risk of worse outcomes than those who remain at home. All the studies in Maclean et al.'s review were carried out in the USA, Sweden or Portugal. The English findings suggesting positive outcomes from care must be regarded as tentative in this context, particularly in the light of the continued poor figures for care leavers' access to higher education. Nonetheless, the policies of the past 15 or so years have resulted in some narrowing of the education 'gap' at school level, and there are some grounds for cautious optimism. In this final chapter I review the key findings of the study that has been the focus of this book; evaluate its contribution to the empirical research literature and to theoretical framings of the responsibilities of the state to the children for whom it has assumed responsibility, particularly as they approach and attain legal adulthood; consider fruitful directions for further research in this area; and assess the implications of the findings in the international context for legislation, policy and practice affecting this small cohort of disadvantaged young people who have a particular claim on the state to safeguard and promote their welfare.

The key findings of the CLET study

In common with the vast majority of the literature in this relatively young area of research, the study is situated in a single national context characterised by a particular social welfare regime and idiosyncratic child protection system. Interpreting the relevance of findings from such a study to other national contexts is notoriously problematic and should be undertaken with caution. Yet English policy on the education of children in care and on their transition to adulthood is worthy of consideration for three primary reasons. First, there has been sustained policy attention to these issues since the turn of the 21st century. Second, there is some evidence that outcomes for English care leavers are improving and that young people age out of care with better prospects than they might otherwise have had (Sebba et al., 2015). Third, the unique status of the English system, which in many respects stands between the social democratic welfare approaches of mainland Europe and Scandinavia and the liberal or neoliberal regimes of the US and other Anglophone countries make it a good case study through which to interrogate key issues of international concern.

There are inherent complexities in researching populations as small, diverse and potentially vulnerable as care leavers. Most young people in care carry significant emotional burdens arising from their pre-care experiences. These are likely to be exacerbated for those entering care late, often after many years of maltreatment, who may also have considerable educational deficits to overcome. A large proportion of these young people have mental health difficulties (Ford et al., 2007; Dubois-Comtois et al., 2015; Greger et al., 2015), which may be exacerbated as they make the transition from care to independent living (Stein and Dumaret, 2011). The methodological implications of this are discussed in Appendix 1, and I will not repeat them here, save to acknowledge that although the sample may well be regarded as no more than opportunistic (see Barnard and Barlow, 2003), the diversity and characteristics of the young people participating do in many respects mirror those in the care population generally, including, for example, the fact that one-third of the cohort was NEET at the end of the study. It should also be borne in mind that the study was not able to take issues relating to young people's mental health directly into account in the analysis.

A particular strength of the study is its longitudinal design. By meeting with young people each year where possible, I was not only able to follow their educational and care experiences over time, but I was able to see directly and to discuss with them the consequences of decisions that they had made in the light of hindsight. I was also able to develop a research relationship with some which enabled them to be more forthcoming with me in the third round of interviews than they were in the first, enhancing the confidence that can be placed in the findings.

It is reassuring that of the 17 young people who participated in the second year of the fieldwork, all considered that being in care had improved their educational outcomes and opportunities, and all but Imogen were clear that removal into state care was the right decision for them. For a number of participants (particularly Riley, who was very clear in his view), it is likely that entry into care at an earlier age would have reduced the disadvantages they faced upon entry and enhanced their prospects as they approached adulthood. The most significant findings in relation to young people's educational progress are reviewed briefly below, followed by consideration of the implications of the findings relating to young people's care experiences for their educational experiences and life outcomes.

From 'low expectations' to 'pushy parents'?

Contrary to earlier literature which is consonant with research internationally, suggesting that professionals and carers held unacceptably low expectations of children's educational potential, this study suggests that the English reforms of this century have served to ensure that education is high on the agenda for most teachers, social workers and carers. It is also clear that the young people themselves placed a high value on education and were acutely aware of the significance of qualifications in the adult world they were about to enter. Virtual heads, designated teachers and young people all appeared to accord particular status to entry to university and, from the evidence of young people such as Jacinda, this was the case in relation to some carers as well. However, if the proportion of young people with a realistic ambition to attend university in this study is an accurate reflection of the wider care population, then arguably we should have expected an increase in university entrants from a care background in the years immediately following the study. Statistical data collection has changed since the study concluded in some respects, but data from 2014–2016 suggest incremental increases, from 6 to 7 per cent of 19-year-old care leavers in higher education and from seven to eight per cent of those aged 19–21 (DfE/NS, 2016a). These rates are still very much lower than the proportion of young people entering university by age 19 in the general population, which stood at 43 per cent for England in 2016 (UCAS, 2016). However, this figure masks that fact that only 16.1 per cent of young people from a lower income background entered university in 2016 – a record high for the sector – as well as much lower entry rates for men than women and considerably lower entry rates for White young people compared with other ethnic groups (UCAS, 2016). These patterns are a reminder that the care leaver population serves as a prism for the study of disadvantage, in which patterns observable in disadvantaged groups more generally are magnified, the conclusion from which must be that discriminatory effects cannot be eliminated entirely by group-specific policies but requires addressing wider issues of structural inequality.

However, the study also suggests that efforts to address the attainment gap, coupled with target-driven policies such as measurement of local authorities' success in terms of numbers of university entrants, may serve not only to divert attention from those who are in danger of 'falling out of everything' (Mr Brook) in favour of the most educationally 'successful' young people, but may also result in a tendency for schools to promote unrealistic expectations, resulting in inevitable disappointment and the need for young people to be 'let down gently' (Mr Brown). These issues also, of course, apply more widely and appear to reflect a culture in which vocational courses are regarded as inferior to more 'academic' studies. A more detailed discussion is beyond the scope of this book, but such questions are highly topical in light of the recent attempts to scale up and to regulate apprenticeship-based learning in England, and wider questions about the implications of an ever-expanding higher education sector internationally in an era of ongoing economic uncertainty. A focus on the individual needs and aspirations of young people in place of a 'one-size-fits-all' measure of success is key to enhancing young people's future prospects in a way which respects their chosen life course rather than serves the evaluation needs of their corporate parent. The potential conflict between the political pressures on corporate parents and their duties to the individual young people for whose upbringing they are responsible is a theme which permeated the CLET study and is reviewed further in other contexts below.

Incentivising attainment or punishing vulnerability?

A pernicious effect of some policy drivers in England and some other nations lies in the way in which the most vulnerable young people – often conceptualised as the most troublesome – are afforded the least support. Systems which measure outcomes by the proportion of children attaining certain target grades inevitably incentivise work with those within reach of the target and render assistance to those who cannot attain that standard within the available timeframe less attractive to professional investment. There is evidence from this study that educationally successful young people may be privileged in other ways by their corporate parent, such as through the continued support of fully-qualified social workers being available only to prospective university students and by the linking of priority for available accommodation to college attendance, as well as the additional financial support they receive while studying. Such measures serve to reinforce the distinction Goldson (2002) calls the '"deserving"–"undeserving" schism' and are likely to result in polarised outcomes at the individual level, where high-achievers are lauded and supported and young people who are struggling, such as Niall, are further marginalised and stigmatised. This is reflected in Tables 7.2–7.4, in which young people participating in the CLET study are designated into Stein's categories of 'Moving On', 'Survivors' and 'Strugglers' (Stein, 2012). The conclusions of the CLET study in this regard were echoed in the findings of a survey of 100 care leavers by the Centre for Social Justice (2014: 4), which concluded that despite genuine advances for care leavers in general, the 'vast majority of spending and support' has been targeted at 'better-off' young people, primarily those in stable foster placements and who continue in education, at cost to those who have not benefited from such targeted support. The extension of the support originally provided through the Children and Young Persons Act 2008 only for care leavers who continue in education, to all care leavers aged up to age 25 by the Children and Social Work Act 2017 (similar to provision in Scotland for support to the age of 26 under the Children and Young People (Scotland)

Act 2014) marks a significant change of heart in English policy, and it will be important to consider its effect in the coming years.

The 16-plus transition

Decisions that young people make about their educational and career pathways post-16 are critical ones for their future prospects, and again this transition was one that was much smoother and easier for young people already doing well. This may be in part because children in care in England are entitled to preferential treatment in school admissions processes and are thereby able to access schools with good academic results. Such schools are likely to have selection criteria for entry to their sixth forms, enabling only those who perform well at 16 to continue in the same school to 18. For those who do not meet the entry criteria to remain in their school beyond GCSEs, or who choose to transfer to college, it appears that this transition is often problematic. The decision as to whether young people will be best served by remaining in school or moving to FE college is very much an individual one. However, there are clear advantages for this cohort in remaining in a familiar and supportive environment, particularly in the context of the concurrent care transitions which young people are likely to be negotiating.

There is limited research in this area internationally, but in the English context, limited support and flexibility at FE colleges appear on the evidence of the CLET study to exacerbate the challenges faced by young people in settling at college. It is clear, however, that many young people have not realised their academic potential by the age of 16, and it is imperative that young people are afforded a 'second chance' to make up any educational deficit they carry as a consequence of their pre-care and/or in-care experiences beyond that age. Government policy aimed at ensuring that young people lacking basic skills are required to study maths and English beyond the age of 16 appears sensible. However, current policy discourages schools from offering a broad-based curriculum in a comprehensive sixth form. There may be a risk that compulsory education or training to the age of 18 will exacerbate the development of a two-tier system, in which FE colleges serve young people taking vocational routes, which are considered to be of lower status, and school sixth forms focus on higher status and more academic pathways (see e.g. Ainley, 2013; Meschi et al., 2014). Similar concerns exist in a broader context in nations in which young people are directed into vocational or academic pathways at a relatively young age. Consideration should be given to allowing care leavers priority admission to the college of their choice, to minimise further disruption and ensure that they are able to access high quality educational provision and a supportive environment. It appears that there may be considerable scope in some local authorities for improvement of retention rates for care leavers attending further education colleges through greater collaboration between virtual schools and designated staff in colleges.

Supporting children in school and beyond

Schools and colleges face a difficult balancing act in supporting older children in care. This research highlights two key tensions. The first relates to the inherent conflict between, on the one hand, pressure on institutions to demonstrate high levels of academic attainment by pupils in a competitive educational 'market' and, on the other, the pastoral needs of young people with disrupted care and educational histories who are likely to present with significant behavioural difficulties and for the most part are less likely to contribute to the perceived success of the institution. Although the use of senior members of staff in the post of designated teacher has the potential advantage of providing a powerful advocate for children in care within the school environment, this conflict may be particularly acute for professionals who are ambitious to progress in their career, who may feel reluctant to challenge their head-teacher. While professional participants in this study all demonstrated an admirably robust approach to their advocacy role, it is clear from the high proportion of young people participating in the study who had been excluded from mainstream school that not all schools honour the expectations that exclusion is an absolute last resort for children in care and that schools continue to support excluded young people to return to school thereafter.

Further, where the post-holder is a member of the senior management team, it is inevitable that young people will perceive them as less approachable and may avoid contact as much as possible, as being likely to draw attention to their care status within school. The model in this study used by Fairfields School of an experienced, senior and highly respected but semi-retired member of staff with no further ambitions and with an exclusively pastoral role in the school appeared to be particularly successful. Other schools had made creative use of administrative staff such as attendance officers, but post-holders in such roles are unlikely to be able to offer the authority of more senior members of staff and add an additional layer of communication. Comparative research on models of support systems in schools and colleges internationally could offer greater illumination of the attributes of successful mechanisms and professionals.

The second tension arises from the interdependence of care and education (Berridge, 2007; Jackson, 2010). The importance of school in providing a normalising environment in which children can detach themselves from their care status (Gilligan, 2000; Martin and Jackson, 2002; Cameron, 2007) should not be underestimated but may be undermined by an overemphasis on children's social care status within school. Young people identify a need for consistent and trusted sources of support and continue to report that these are rarely accessed through social services. Designated teachers may provide children in care with a consistent professional to advise and support them in their educational career, but teachers cannot – and should not – substitute for professional social workers.

This study suggests that, while designated teachers appear to be a valuable resource in many respects, their relative lack of involvement in management of young people's transitions to other institutions at 16-plus may be a weakness. In some instances, this appeared to be associated with young people's move to the leaving care team and a perception by designated teachers that arrangements were the concern of that team and not of the school. There was also some evidence to suggest that relations between schools and colleges were perceived as competitive and/or that further education colleges were reluctant to liaise with schools or were poorly equipped to do so. These difficulties reflect perennial observations as to the challenges in three areas: first, joint working across disciplinary boundaries such as education and social care; second, overcoming the introduction of competition in educational provision; and third, effecting smooth educational transitions for children in care. In some cases, providers of alternative provision appeared to be more focused and engaged in actively managing this transition on behalf of young people who needed high levels of support in further education, and mainstream schools might usefully develop similar arrangements.

The virtual head model appears to be a potentially valuable one in enabling corporate parents to fulfil their statutory duty to promote the educational attainment of children in care. At the time of the study, there was mixed provision of schools that operated under the oversight of their local authority, which was also responsible for social care provision in the local area, and those which enjoyed greater independence. On the evidence presented here, virtual schools can promote communication and co-operation between social care and education, ensure that the education of children in care is given high priority within both arenas and facilitate the translation of corporate parenting policy into individual attention to the unique needs of young people. A significant advantage of the virtual school system was evidenced in enhanced communication to schools regarding the background and needs of new entrants into care. Another benefit was the ability of virtual heads to work constructively with schools, to challenge them and hold them to account, as well as to support social workers to do so (see also Ofsted, 2012), attributed by participants to their senior status and educational backgrounds. Where their remit extends into adulthood, virtual schools may provide invaluable continuity through educational and social care transitions. While local arrangements will vary greatly across and within nations, the findings demonstrate the benefits of systems which facilitate close co-operation between social care and education and the potential disadvantages of a marketised education system in which schools and colleges compete with one another and are focused on demonstrating success through decontextualised markers of educational attainment.

The interdependence of educational outcomes and
young people's experiences in care

One of the strongest and most disappointing findings from young people's accounts of their experiences in care is that despite repeated exhortations in the literature internationally for steps to be taken to address the harm arising from high turnover and caseloads of social workers, young people still reported experiencing poor continuity of social work and were unable to develop meaningful and trusting relationships with the professionals most directly responsible for their welfare. Moreover, no participants in the CLET study identified individuals whom they regarded as supportive adults outside of their foster care or school environment who would be available to them during their transition out of care: while some designated teachers, notably Mr Brown, provided such a model, they would not be available after young people left school. Nor did young people refer to long-term informal relationships of the sort identified in the resilience literature (e.g. Gilligan, 2008) as valuable during life transitions, either spontaneously or in answer to questions about supportive individuals in their lives. Coupled with the pervasiveness of poor quality placements, unhappiness in placements and/or multiple disruptions in placements, this led to a degree of instability in participants' personal lives directly associated with their experiences in care. Focal theory helps to account for the way in which young people's educational progress may easily be derailed by disruption in their care, even without taking into account the practical consequences, such as disrupted educational placements, that might result from such events.

Echoing the findings of the Care Inquiry (The Care Inquiry, 2013), the CLET study suggests that there is an urgent need to refocus attention on care leavers' personal relationships with significant adults. In particular, consideration needs to be given to how the legal parent of children in care can provide the level of individual care and attention that most children take for granted from their birth parents. Over 30 years ago, Freeman (1983: 168) wrote '[t]here is no way in which one can equate flesh and blood parents with legal parents in a care setting', citing in particular bureaucratic decision-making by people unacquainted with the children for whom they are responsible and the prevalence of poorly paid workers in residential care homes. While roughly three-quarters of children in care are now cared for in foster-placements in England, too few young people in this study enjoyed a genuinely warm and close relationship with their carers akin to that of family life at its best, and it is tempting to conclude that little has changed in children's lived experience of care.

The English government responded to concerns about the nature of corporate parenting by the introduction of 'Corporate Parenting Principles' in section 1 of the Children and Social Work Act 2017, which requires local authorities, when carrying out their functions with regard to children in care or care leavers under the age of 25 to:

> have regard to the need—(a) to act in the best interests, and promote the physical and mental health and well-being, of those children and young people; (b) to encourage those children and young people to express their views, wishes and feelings; (c) to take into account the views, wishes and feelings of those children and young people; (d) to help those children and young people gain access to, and make the best use of, services provided by the local authority and its relevant partners; (e) to promote high aspirations, and seek to secure the best outcomes, for those children and young people; (f) for those children and young people to be safe, and for stability in their home lives, relationships and education or work; (g) to prepare those children and young people for adulthood and independent living.

This legislation also boosts the requirements for local authorities to provide and publish information about services for care leavers, including those relating to their health and well-being, relationships and participation in society, as well as their education and training, employment and accommodation. While it is reassuring to see a clear recognition of the significance of relationships and participation in society in legislation, such acknowledgement on its own is unlikely to make a significant difference to outcomes for care leavers, given the many challenges.

In the English context, it would be valuable to explore the way in which the devolution of greater decision-making powers to carers operates and whether it has the desired effect of making children feel more 'at home' in their placements. Consideration should be given to the vesting of parental responsibility in an individual where possible and agreeable to the child themselves. Alternative models might fall short of investing a named person with legal parental responsibility but promote long-term relationships between children and adults whom they know or may come to know well. English-speaking nations would do well to consider what can be learnt from the way in which the social pedagogic approach successfully marries the professional and the personal to fulfil children's needs for parental care as well as parental responsibility.

In the CLET study, feelings of rejection and/or loss with regard to relationships with birth parents were acute for many participants. The extent to which relationships with their birth parents were a source of distress and a preoccupation for young people reflects the findings of other research, including Sinclair et al. (2005) and Biehal et al. (2010). Research has identified the risks involved in children becoming caught up in potentially damaging family dynamics through contact with their birth families as well as the importance of social work support for contact to their birth family for children in long-term placements (Sen and Broadhurst, 2011). However, consideration of the focal model may shift attention to issues of timeliness and in particular the importance of establishing patterns of high quality contact as early as possible wherever it is safe to do so, and where it is not, ensuring the child is given appropriate explanations of that decision (Sen and Broadhurst, 2011).

The CLET study also found that, contrary to the statutory requirement that siblings should be placed together unless impracticable (Children Act s22C(8)), but consistent with the literature (Sen and Broadhurst, 2011), many young people were placed apart from their siblings either on entry into care or as circumstances changed at later dates. While some of these changes may have been unavoidable, they were not only a source of distress to young people, they also inflicted further significant life changes over the course of the study on young people already burdened by multiple changes. More research is needed into contact with siblings for children in out-of-home care (Sen and Broadhurst, 2011), particularly in the context of the complex family structures described by many participants in this study. Where young people have had limited or no contact with members of their birth family when they are under 18, more attention could be paid to preparatory counselling and advice for young people before they seek to reestablish these relationships.

Theorising care leavers' transitions

In 2006, Stein (2006b) drew attention to the a-theoretical nature of much of the research on the experiences of and outcomes for young people ageing out of care. Stein himself suggested use of attachment theory, resilience theory and the focal model of adolescence as potential frameworks, but the response to Stein's call for more attention to theoretical insights has been somewhat muted. Although there has been some use of the literature on attachment 'state of mind' in adolescence in order to understand care leavers' relationship difficulties in early adulthood, this area remains relatively poorly understood. In the last decade researchers concerned with the care population have increasingly used a resilience framework, in part to enable movement away from a deficit model of social care recipients towards focusing on individual strengths and personal agency, both of which may be especially pertinent in relation to adolescents as they develop their adult identities and become increasingly autonomous. Application of Stein's categorisation of care leavers as 'Moving On', 'Survivors' and 'Strugglers' (2012), derived from resilience theory, has in this study drawn attention to the way in which policies designed to incentivise young people to pursue further and higher education privilege those who are already comparatively well-equipped to succeed in adult life. Combining insights from the focal model of adolescence and resilience theory highlights the need to turn policy on its head to ensure that young people are not punished for their inability to address multiple challenges in their personal lives and education within the timeframes dictated by state institutions.

The focal model of adolescence has particular resonance for the lives of young people who have experienced disruption and trauma in or shortly before adolescence and is especially powerful in explaining the needs of late entrants into care. Although it is not free from criticism and is relatively underdeveloped in the literature, it offers a powerful explanation for the particular difficulties faced by care leavers in their transition to adulthood. Stein has described this process as 'accelerated and compressed' (Stein, 2006a: 274), to capture the way in which care leavers generally become independent at an earlier age than their peers, after a shorter transition period and with little or no opportunity to return 'home' should they encounter difficulties. Education and social care systems both impose enforced transitions upon young people for whom the developmental tasks of adolescence are more problematic than for those growing up within their birth families and who may concurrently be grappling with significant personal challenges, including emotional trauma and educational deficits. Consequently, care leavers are likely to have limited control over the way in which they manage the multiple issues arising in adolescence. They are likely to need more time than their peers to make a successful transition to independent adulthood, yet they tend to be catapulted into, and/or actively choose, independence at an earlier age. The focal model of adolescence explains the need for the creation of more normative transitions for young people leaving care (Stein, 2006a). Recent developments in many nations have acknowledged this by allowing some children to remain in placements beyond the age of legal majority and make a gradual transition to independent living. It will be important for research to evaluate how successful such schemes are, particularly with regard to young people whose life experiences have induced strong feelings of self-reliance.

My own concern as a former practitioner, as a children's rights advocate, and indeed as a parent, lies with the care and upbringing of each *individual* child. Population-level statistics all too easily mask the personal fates of the most disadvantaged members of a cohort whose prospects may be worsened by policies that appear effective in increasing outcomes for the group as a whole. This study has attempted to demonstrate that Coleman's focal model of adolescence and a children's rights perspective can both illuminate the way in which policy initiatives may serve to privilege the child that achieves at an apparent cost to the child who might be regarded as less of a credit to his or her corporate parent, exposing the inherent injustice in incentive-driven policies. I have also argued that a rights-based analysis provides the most illuminating means to assess how well-equipped individual young people are to exercise autonomy in adulthood. Young people's own perspectives have therefore been foregrounded in the analysis in order to avoid the potential pitfalls associated with relying on the interpretation of professionals or other adults as to what is considered to be in a child's best interests or what a young person plans for their future.

Research in this area has generally remained welfare-oriented and rooted in social care discourses rather than underpinned by frameworks of rights. This circumstance may be a reflection of child and family social work itself, which has tended to be needs-based and to overlook considerations of children's agency, competence and rights (Goodyear, 2013). Although greater attention has been paid to children's participation rights in social care work in English legislation and policy in recent years, Broadhurst et al. (2009: 251) conclude that children's rights in general did not 'appear to fit easily' with the political priorities of the New Labour administration. And more recently, the rhetoric of the Conservative and Liberal Democrat Coalition (2010–2015) and Conservative (2015-) Governments has tended to focus on strengthening families rather than on the rights of children as individuals, perhaps reflecting discourse in the US, where there is a strong tradition of 'parents' rights' rhetoric (see e.g. Shulman (2014) for a critique of the Constitutional underpinnings of this tradition). Yet over 25 years after the introduction of the United Nations Convention on the Rights of the Child (UNCRC) (UNGA, 1989), now ratified by every country in the world save the US, a framework of children's rights is becoming the dominant international discourse in the conceptualisation and measurement of national responses to issues pertaining to child well-being. Arguably, greater use of analysis using a rights framework is overdue.

I have drawn upon Hollingsworth's theory of 'foundational rights' to present a richer understanding of the conditions required for the exercise of 'full' autonomy. The value of Hollingsworth's conceptualisation of foundational rights lies particularly in its movement beyond material or skills-based aspects of autonomy to an incorporation of relational factors in the development of autonomy, providing a powerful response to the criticisms of commentators such as Smith (2009) that rights-based frameworks overlook the significance of relationships and social context within care work. There is much conceptual work to be done in relation to the notion of foundational rights, but future work drawing on young people's own understanding of their autonomy and the potential relationship between self-reliance and the development of 'full' autonomy would be valuable. Research could usefully build on the concept of foundational rights in order to develop more concrete suggestions as to the nature and extent of the state's responsibilities in all areas of the lives of children for whom the state has seized parental responsibility. Such work should be underpinned by an expectation first, that children of the state are entitled not just to a similar level of 'parental' support as those who remain in the care of their birth parents, but to reparation for the harm they have suffered; and second, that they are likely to retain a degree of dependence on parental support for many years after they attain legal adulthood.

Considering the prospects of young people ageing out of care through the lens of foundational rights brings into focus the particular 'assets' required by young people as they approach legal adulthood. In particular, accounts of autonomy as a relational concept reinforce the argument as to the significance of personal relationships with supportive and caring adults in the lives of young people ageing out of care. While the focus of attention on social pedagogy has primarily been in early years and residential care work, there is potential synergy between foundational rights theory and the principles of social pedagogy. The concern of social pedagogy with participatory principles, equality, relational and emotional development, and young people's emerging citizenship and engagement in society may provide a practical framework through which to work consciously towards the realisation of young people's foundational rights.

Conclusion

Across economically advanced nations, care leavers remain one of the most disadvantaged groups in society. Yet recent statistics and research showing a narrowing gap between the educational attainment of children in care and that of their peers in response to targeted policies attest to the fact that poor educational outcomes are not inevitable for this group of young people. Indeed, such improvements appear to confirm that state care has not previously succeeded in maximising the opportunities of this group to achieve their potential, suggesting a universal failure on behalf of the state in discharging its reparatory responsibility towards the children entrusted to its care. Although it is important to bear in mind that some of these young people, such as Ollie in this study, are in care for reasons which preclude them from meeting population-level targets for attainment, the gap remains wide, suggesting that there remains much work to be done. While focused support from within the educational estate, such as the introduction of designated teachers in English schools, has a valuable contribution to make in improving the educational attainment of children in care, three related points arise from the CLET study.

The first concerns evidence that young people's opportunities in the educational arena may be undermined by failings in the social care estate. The corporate parent must act not only as an educated and informed parent but also as a caring parent if it is to maximize the life chances of the children for whom it holds responsibility. International evidence demonstrates that for the most vulnerable children, close, stable and supportive adult relationships may be especially challenging to achieve but are likely to be a prerequisite for full engagement in learning. Cross-national comparison suggests a range of ways in which the parent state attempts to compensate for the absence of 'flesh and blood' parents, often with limited success. Placement instability has proven difficult to address, and it may be time for a more imaginative approach, such as one which draws on the principles of social pedagogy.

The second relates to management of transition points within young people's care and education trajectories: such moments may become 'turning-points' for better or worse, to use the language of the resilience literature. It was apparent that the period of young people's lives covered by the study was regarded by professionals as critical to their long-term success and that there were both opportunities and particular difficulties associated with the transition to further education for young people in care. Professional participants identified a number of characteristics of the care population which created particular challenges in ensuring a successful educational transition at 16, especially the high proportion of late entrants into care and behavioural issues. While the age of this particular transition (and/or that to higher education, vocational training or employment) may vary from country to country, the insights provided by this study as to the need for professionals to be sensitive to and take advantage of both transition points that might provide either opportunities or challenges to young people and young people's individual developmental trajectories, apply universally. In particular, it is imperative that universal transition points are utilized as opportunities for a reappraisal and fresh start for young people outside mainstream schooling or who have become disengaged from education. Young people who have not achieved academically by a predetermined age should not be 'written off' or irrevocably directed into less prestigious career trajectories, and their corporate parent should provide continued support for its children to continue to develop their full academic potential.

The final point relates to the importance of sustained support for young people beyond 16 and into emerging adulthood: care leavers should be entitled to the seamless and personal support typically available to their peers from their birth or adoptive parents. Perhaps most importantly, and also in line with the natural expectations society makes of birth parents, the corporate parent must be able to effect a personalized response to the needs of each individual child in its care and recognize that the most vulnerable children are entitled to the highest level of support for the longest period of time. If care leavers are to develop their capabilities to the extent that will enable their foundational rights to be fulfilled, the corporate parent must accept that reparatory responsibility imports an ongoing parental role in the lives of young people until such time as they are able to overcome the consequences of the harm they have suffered. Only then will care leavers be able to take their place in society as fully autonomous citizens.

Appendix 1
Methodology

The study methodology

There are particular methodological challenges in carrying out research involving care leavers, arising from the vulnerability of the participants; the size, mobility and geographical spread of the population; and their tendency to be socially excluded and stigmatised (Wigfall and Cameron, 2006). A qualitative research strategy was employed to enable a detailed exploration of young people's perspectives in the context of intricate lives in which personal and educational strands were interdependent (Trinder, 1996).

The research questions and methods for this study built on those of a pilot study involving in-depth semi-structured interviews with seven care leavers aged 16 to 20 (Driscoll, 2011, 2013a), expanding on the earlier study by capturing the perspectives of designated teachers and virtual school heads as well as a larger number of young people and by adopting a longitudinal design. The study was designed to recruit approximately 20 young people, to interview them about their educational experiences and plans at age 15–16 and then to re-interview as many as possible in each of the following two academic years, in the expectation of a high level of disengagement as the study progressed. The designated teachers (in schools) and safeguarding officers (in further educational colleges for young people aged 16 and over) of the young people participating in the study were also invited to participate through an interview about their wider experience of their role in supporting young people in school or college. Two local authorities agreed to support the research through their 'virtual schools' (units within local authorities with responsibility for all children in care of school age in that local authority area). Ethical approval was gained from the Association of Directors of Children's Services (ADCS) in order to access additional cases outside those local authorities, for example where young people in the care of one authority were in school in another. Approval was also obtained from the committee for 'high risk' research projects (SSHL RESC)[1] at my university.

This mode of access helped to ensure that very vulnerable young people were not approached. It also arose from a desire to achieve a sample that, if not 'representative' of the care population, at least would reflect its diversity.

The two local authorities engaged in the research, identified by the fictitious names Riversmeet (virtual head Mr Brook) and Stonycross (virtual head Ms Mason) are located in urban areas with ethnically diverse populations of over 300,000 (Greater London Authority Intelligence Unit, 2012). Nonetheless, selection and access arrangements affected the recruitment of young people to the study, as reported in similar studies involving vulnerable children and young people (see, for example Barnard and Barlow, 2003). In particular, because access and informed consent arrangements involved school head-teachers and designated teachers as well as children's social care managers and social workers, there were layers of opportunity for professionals to decline participation on behalf of young people, including on the basis of their own assessment of the young person's vulnerability.

'Gatekeepers' such as teachers have an important role in protecting children and young people from potential harm (Masson, 2000), but they may also be inclined to 'err on the side of caution' where vulnerable children are concerned (Cree et al., 2002: 50). In a study of researchers working with children and young people, Heath et al. (2007) concluded that in institutions such as schools which separate children from society as a whole there is a tendency to construct young people as incompetent to make decisions for themselves, resulting in the conflation of the right to grant access with the right to consent. In this study, social workers generally appeared willing to allow young people more autonomy than did their teachers, perhaps reflecting differences in professional roles and relationships with children. Gatekeepers may also 'use their position to censor children and young people' (Masson, 2000: 36), including to exclude young people who might not behave conformably (Crow et al., 2006). In a review of research studies involving adopted or fostered children, Murray (2005) describes gatekeeping practice as reflecting 'the pervasiveness of a protectionist model of children and young people over a citizen-with-rights model' (64), although in that review, as in this study, it is clear that in many cases professionals had good reason for taking such a stance. In the case of children in care, multiple consent requirements may also contribute to a pattern of over-protection that operates to exclude such young people from making decisions for themselves and thereby denies them the opportunity to develop the necessary competencies for autonomous adulthood (Leeson, 2007).

Additionally, decisions made in managing the study's feasibility inevitably limited its scope. First, the study design only included professionals from an education background. Ideally, to obtain a full picture of a young person's progress and support networks, the study would have included perspectives from social workers and from foster carers. However, although social workers exercise parental responsibility for children in care on behalf of the local authority corporate parent, their contribution was of less relevance to this study; there is often a fast turnover of staff which may limit the input they would be able to provide, and young people often have a difficult relationship with social care staff, which might have affected their willingness to speak with me in the knowledge that their social worker would also be speaking about them. Similarly, young people might have felt the inclusion of their foster carer's views to be intrusive, whereas their designated teacher would usually be a senior member of school staff who would know them less well as individuals and be associated with their educational rather than personal lives. Second, I did not explore issues of mental health and was therefore only aware of mental or emotional health issues raised by young people themselves, which I did not consider it ethical to pursue further given the focus of the study and my own lack of expertise in that area. The high level of need and difficulties in accessing mental health services (Mooney et al., 2009) both remain significant concerns for this group which are likely to impact on their educational experiences and attainment and should be borne in mind, particularly in relation to accounts of challenging behaviour.

In total, 21 young people participated in the study, nine of whom were interviewed in all three years. 18 young people took part in the first year of the study, 17 in the second and 10 in the third, making a total of 45 interviews. 12 designated teachers, seven in mainstream schools and five in alternative provision; three officers in further education colleges with responsibility for care leavers; and five professionals from local authority virtual schools also participated. In all, therefore, 65 interviews were conducted. Findings are presented with acknowledgement that the professionals who participated are not necessarily representative of all post-holders. Teachers agreeing to take part in a study such as this are likely to be highly motivated by the challenges of the role and particularly reflexive in their professional practice. Care leavers are a diverse group and participants were interviewed during a period of their lives which is one of particularly rapid development and change.

Despite the difficulties in access, the 21 young people participating in the project reflected the constituency of young people in care reasonably well. There were 12 boys (57 per cent) and 9 girls (43 per cent), close to the gender ratio of 56 per cent male and 44 per cent female in the care population nationally at the time the fieldwork commenced (DfE/NS, 2011). Only nine were white British, with the sample reflecting the diverse populations of the geographical areas in which the participants lived. Of the 18 whose care status was known, 10 (56 per cent) were the subject of compulsory care orders, compared with 60 per cent in the care population as a whole in England, and seven were voluntarily accommodated, compared with 31 per cent of all children in care. One had been remanded into care in youth justice proceedings. As can be seen from Table A.1, 13 of the young people attended mainstream schools (marked M) at the start of the study, three were in Pupil Referral Units (PRUs) (for children excluded from school), and two attended special schools (S) (catering for children with significant disabilities or Special Educational Needs, including social, emotional and behavioural needs). Three (accessed through the charitable organisation by which they were accommodated) were not in education at all.

Table A.1 Young participants

Name[1] (gender)	Ethnicity	Into care	School Year 11	Special needs etc.
Adam (M)	White	Year 5	Woodhall M	
Bashir (M)	Asian DLR[2]	Year 8	Woodhall M	EAL
Callum (M)	White	End Year 7	Woodhall M	Offending
Devora (F)	White	Year 9	Ravenscourt M	Orphan
Elliott (M)	Mixed	Year 7	Fairfields M	
Farouk (M)	Asian UASC[3]	Year 7	King's M	EAL
Gilroy (M)	Mixed	End Year 7	Clifton M	Offending, speech impediment
Habib (M)	Asian refugee	Year 5	PRU	EAL, ADHD
Imogen (F)	Black	Year 4	Queen's M	
Jacinda (F)	Mixed	Year 1	Queen's M	
Kayla (F)	Black	Year 1	Garden House M	
Luis (M)	Mixed	Year 2	The Grove S (EBD)	Long-term support
Michael (M)	White	Age 4	Meadowpond M	Asperger's Syndrome SEN
Niall (M)	White	Year 8	Redhouse PRU	Literacy SEN
Ollie (M)	White	?	Stonehouse S	Physical and learning disabilities SEN
Priya (F)	Asian	Age 13 (Year 8/9)	M	Teenage mother
Qadira (F)	Black	Age 12/13 (Year 7/8)	Not in school (PRU)	Secure care home
Riley (M)	White	Age 15 (Year 10/11)	Seaview PRU	Offending
Sofia (F)	Black/mixed UASC[3]	Age 16 (Year 11)	Fairfields M	EAL
Tasmin (F)	White	Age 8	Fairfields M	
Unity (F)	White	Age 11	Not in school (PRU)	Secure unit 4 times

1 All names are pseudonyms to protect the identity of participants and schools.
2 DLR = Discretionary Leave to Remain.
3 UASC = Unaccompanied Asylum-Seeking Child.

It is difficult to draw conclusions about any distinctions between young people who agreed to participate and those that declined because in many cases the invitation to participate was not passed on by the school, and in others the school considered that participation was not appropriate. Some designated teachers felt that the exercise would be of benefit to the young person in question and therefore took pains to encourage their participation. It is reasonable to speculate that those who participated were likely to be

Table A.2 Interviews undertaken over the three years of the CLET study

Name[1] (gender)	Year 11	Year 12	Year 13	No. of interviews
Adam (M)	✓	✓	✓	3
Bashir (M)	✓	✓	✓	3
Callum (M)	✓	✓	✓	3
Devora (F)	✓	✓	✓	3
Elliott (M)	✓	—	—	1
Farouk (M)	✓	✓	—	2
Gilroy (M)	✓	✓	—	2
Habib (M)	✓	✓	✓	3
Imogen (F)	✓	✓	✓	3
Jacinda (F)	✓	✓	✓	3
Kayla (F)	✓	✓	✓	3
Luis (M)	✓	✓	—	2
Michael (M)	✓	—	—	1
Niall (M)	✓	—	—	1
Ollie (M)	✓	✓	—	2
Priya (F)	—	✓	—	1
Qadira (F)	✓	✓	✓	3
Riley (M)	—	✓	✓	2
Sofia (F)	✓	—	—	1
Tasmin (F)	✓	✓	—	2
Unity (F)	—	✓	—	1
Total	18	17	10	45

1 All names are pseudonyms to protect the identity of participants.

more conscious of the importance of education to their future life prospects and willing to engage at least with some professionals. It was not possible to meet with all of the young people each year. Table A.2 shows the pattern of interviews carried out. Where participants did not take part in follow-up interviews it was often the case that they were difficult to access because they had left school and ceased to engage with social workers.

Professional participants

Designated teachers

The teacher participants came from 12 institutions in eight local authorities, comprising seven mainstream schools, including one academy; one private and two maintained special schools; and two alternative providers (or Pupil Referral Units), one maintained and one private. All the mainstream schools included 16-plus provision. The three state-funded, non-mainstream institutions took young people to the age of 16, but the two private institutions included young people up to 17 and 19 respectively. Of the seven mainstream schools, two were faith schools (one Christian and one Jewish), and two were girls' schools. All five of the non-mainstream institutions accepted a mixed intake, although the two private schools had only boys on roll at the time of the research. All the designated teachers interviewed had experience of young people looked after by a number of different local authorities, enabling them to compare practice between local authority areas: Ms Olive dealt with nine different authorities.

The experience of participants in the designated teacher role varied widely. Two were new in the post at the start of that academic year, while the most experienced post-holders in the mainstream schools had been designated teachers for nine and 10 years respectively. Consequently, the number of looked-after children that participants had worked with ranged from three to around 150. Most participants held a senior post within the school hierarchy. Only one was part-time, and he was semi-retired from a senior management position. All had reduced teaching loads or undertook no teaching in light of their additional responsibilities. Of the non-mainstream institutions, the head-teacher took responsibility for children in care in three institutions, and a deputy head in the other two, although the private institutions did not recognise a named designated teacher role as such. All the non-mainstream institutions had higher proportions of looked-after children on roll than the mainstream schools. Therefore, even where the post was not officially designated, staff often had considerable experience and expertise in the education of children in care. Table A.3 summarises the roles and experience of the teacher participants.

Staff in further education colleges

Since there is no statutory or even conventional model for the oversight of care leavers within further education colleges, responsibility is held at different levels and through different roles, and it was difficult to ascertain whom to approach in colleges. At Millbank College, Ms Willow was Learner Services Manager, which included responsibility for the safeguarding team of 10 members of staff. The latter was a relatively new innovation, around five years old, and Ms Willow's background was unconventional, as she explained: 'I'm a mum whose children had a lot of issues... I've got life experience'. Ms Maple at Eastside College had also come into the role because of her wider experience, in this case as a foster carer. At the time of the interview she had only just taken on the additional role of 'designated coach' for looked-after children and teenage parents. Ms Oak at Forest Hill College was the most senior of the three officers in further education colleges, as Director of Learning Services.

The three colleges were at very different stages in the way in which they identified and supported care leavers. Ms Willow was unable to identify the number of care leavers on roll at Millbank College, although the college was in the process of addressing this issue in order to ensure that the 16–19 bursary scheme was appropriately administered. Ms Maple was responsible for 60 young people at Eastside College but stated that this figure had reduced by about a quarter from the start of the academic year to the time of the interview

Table A.3 Designated teacher participants

Name[1] (school)	Post held	Experience No of LAC (time in post)	School profile
Mr Black (Ravenscourt)	Assistant head-teacher	3 (4 years)	Mixed Voluntary Aided faith school
Mr Brown (Woodhall)	Part-time, pastoral leadership role	c150 (10 years)	Mixed Academy
Ms Carmine (Redhouse)	Head	2 (2 years)	Private mixed alternative education provision
Ms Coral (Seaview)	Deputy head	9 (2 years)	Mixed Pupil Referral Unit
Mr Green (Fairfields)	Assistant head-teacher	10/11 (18 months)	Mixed Community school
Mr Grey (Stonehouse)	Head	c140 (28 years)	Mixed special school, learning and behavioural needs
Ms Gold (Queen's)	Assistant head-teacher	7 (5 years)	Girls' Community school
Ms Olive (The Grove)	Head	c70 (7 years)	Private mixed special school, Educational/Behavioural/Social needs
Ms Rose (Garden House)	Inclusion and learning support manager	4 (6 months)	Girls' Community school
Ms Tan (Sunnyhill)	Head of Care	c150 (15 years)	Mixed Community school Educational/Behavioural/Social needs
Ms Teal (Meadowpond)	Inclusion co-ordinator (senior management)	25–30 (9 years)	Mixed Foundation school
Ms White (Clifton)	Inclusion leader, upper school	5 (6 months)	Mixed Voluntary Aided faith school

1 Pseudonyms are used for teachers and schools to maintain anonymity.

Table A.4 Virtual school participants

Name, local authority[1]	Professional experience	Structure	Virtual school time and role	Virtual school
Ms Lea, The Valleys	18/19 years teaching, LA behaviour management adviser	In CLA service, delivered by private company	11 years, virtual head or equivalent. Part-time	Up to age 16. c200 children, high proportion out of borough, 17 staff before cuts
Mr Steel, Ironbridge	25 years teaching, deputy head	In School Improvement Service	2.5 years @.4, lead officer for LAC	Very recently extended to 18, c240 children, c1/6 out of borough, total staff 2 FTE
Mr Brook, Riversmeet	Educational psychologist, trained as teacher	Multi-agency team in LAC services in CSD	3 years @.5, virtual head (but set up multi-agency team 10 years ago)	Extending over 18, c310 children. Staff: Educational psychologist, education officer
Ms Mason, Stonycross	Teaching background, inc. HT 18 years, challenging school	In corporate parenting, in social care	3 years @.4 virtual head	Up to age 16, seeking 18. C 300 children. Staff: 4 people, 2 × .4, including VH, advisory teacher, Educational psychologist
Ms Ford, Wadebridge	Teacher to retirement age, assistant head and designated for child protection and LAC	In multi-disciplinary virtual school leadership team within Education Department	2 years @.4 Consultant teacher, secondary	Up to 18+. 100–110 children. Staff: VH @.1, 2 consultants each @.4, primary and secondary

1 All names are pseudonyms to protect the identity of participants and local authorities.

in early March, which she attributed primarily to non-attendance or young people moving out of the area. Ms Oak at Forest Hill College stated that, of the 4,500 full-time students aged 16 to 18 at the college, 45 (1 per cent) were from care, and that the retention rate that year for that cohort was 90 per cent.

Virtual school heads and staff

Of the five staff interviewed from virtual schools, three were virtual heads, one was employed as a 'consultant teacher' and the fifth was a secondary senior advisor with responsibility for children in care. Four of the five participants came from urban local authorities: the fifth was employed by an authority in a largely affluent and white middle-class area. Four had extensive teaching experience, one as a head-teacher, one as a deputy head, and one as an assistant head and designated teacher, while the fourth had progressed to the local authority's behaviour management service. The fifth virtual head was an educational psychologist. Table A.4 shows the professional backgrounds of the virtual school staff who participated in the study, together with details of the structural arrangements in their local authority, their experience and the numbers of children for whom they were responsible.

Note

1 Social Science & Public Policy, Humanities and Law Research Ethics Subcommittee.

References

Ahrens, K., DuBois, D., Garrison, M., Spencer, R., Richardson, L. & Lozano, P. 2011. Qualitative exploration of relationships with important non-parental adults in the lives of youth in foster care. *Children and Youth Services Review*, 33(6), 1012–1023.

Ahrens, K., Katon, W., McCarty, C., Richardson, L. & Courtney, M. 2012. Association between childhood sexual abuse and transactional sex in youth aging out of foster care. *Child Abuse & Neglect*, 36(1), 75–80.

Ainley, P. 2013. Education and the reconstitution of social class in England. *Research in Post-Compulsory Education*, 18(1–2), 46–60.

Ainsworth, M., Blehar, M., Waters, E. & Wall, S. 1978. *Patterns of Attachment: A Psychological Study of the Strange Situation*. Hilllsdale, NJ: Lawrence Erlbaum Associates.

Ajayi, S. & Quigley, M. 2006. By degrees: Care leavers in higher education. In: Chase, E., Simon, A. & Jackson, S. (eds.) *In Care and After: A Positive Perspective*. London: Routledge, 63–81.

Albus, S., Greschke, H., Klingler, B., Messmer, H., Micheel, H.-G., Otto, H.-U. & Polutta, A. 2010. *Wirkungsorientierte Jugendhilfe*. Münster, Germany: ISA.

Allen, M. 2003. *Into the Mainstream: Care Leavers Entering Work, Education and Training*. York: Joseph Rowntree Foudation.

Allen, J., McElhaney, K., Land, D., Kuperminc, G., Moore, C., O'Beirne-Kelly, H. & Kilmer, S. 2003. A Secure base in adolescence: Markers of attachment security in the mother–Adolescent relationship. *Child Development*, 74(1), 292–307.

Allen, B. & Vacca, J. 2010. Frequent moving has a negative affect on the school achievement of foster children makes the case for reform. *Children and Youth Services Review*, 32(6), 829–832.

American Psychiatric Association, 2012. *Diagnostic and Statistical Manual of Mental Disorders (DSM) Fifth Edition, DSM-5*. Washington, DC: American Psychiatric Association.

Andersen, S. & Fallesen, P. 2015. Family matters? The effect of kinship care on foster care disruption rates. *Child Abuse & Neglect*, 48, 68–79.

Arnett, J. 2000. Emerging adulthood: A theory of development from the late teens through the twenties. *American Psychologist*, 55(5), 469–480.

Association of Directors of Children's Services (ADCS)/National Consortium for Examination Results/National Association of Virtual School Heads. 2015. *Joint Policy Paper: The Educational Achievement of Children in Care*. Association of

Directors of Children's Services/National Consortium for Examination Results/ National Association of Virtual School Heads.

Atkins, L. 2010. Opportunity and aspiration, or the great deception? The case of 14–19 vocational education. *Power and Education,* 2(3), 253–265.

Atkins, L. 2016. The odyssey: School to work transitions, serendipity and position in the field. *British Journal of Sociology of Education,* 1–12. doi:10.1080/01425692. 2015.1131146.

Baker, K. 2014. *The Skills Mismatch.* London: Edge Foundation.

Ball, S., Maguire, M. & Macrae, S. 2000. *Choice, Pathways and Transitions Post-16: New Youth, New Economies in the Global City.* London: RoutledgeFalmer.

Bankston, C. & Zhou, M. 2002. Being well vs. doing well: Self-esteem and school performance among immigrant and nonimmigrant racial and ethnic groups. *The International Migration Review,* 36(2), 389–415.

Bannink, R., Broeren, S., van de Looij – Jansen, P. & Raat, H. 2013. Associations between parent-adolescent attachment relationship quality, negative life events and mental health. *PLOS One,* 8(11), e80812.

Barnard, M. & Barlow, J. 2003. Discovering parental drug dependence: Silence and disclosure. *Children & Society,* 17(1), 45–56.

Beckett, C., Pinchen, I. & McKeigue, B. 2014. Permanence and 'Permanence': Outcomes of Family Placements. *British Journal of Social Work* 44, 1162–1179.

Bender, K., Yang, J., Ferguson, K. & Thompson, S. 2015. Experiences and needs of homeless youth with a history of foster care. *Children and Youth Services Review,* 55, 222–231.

Bentley, C. 2013. Great Expectations: Supporting "unrealistic" aspirations for children in care. In S. Jackson, *Pathways through Education for Young People in Care: Ideas from Research and Practice.* London: British Association for Adoption and Fostering, 45–52.

Berlin, M., Vinnerljung, B. & Hjern, A. 2011. School performance in primary school and psychosocial problems in young adulthood among care leavers from long term foster care. *Children and Youth Services Review,* 33(12), 2489–2497.

Bernedo, I., Salas, M., Fuentes, M. & García-Martín, M. 2014. Foster children's behavior problems and impulsivity in the family and school context. *Children and Youth Services Review,* 42, 43–49.

Bernedo, I. M., García-Martín, M. A. & Salas, M. D. &. Fuentes, M.J. 2015. Placement stability in non-kinship foster care: Variables associated with placement disruption. *European Journal of Social Work,* 19(6), 917–993.

Berridge, D. 2007. Theory and explanation in child welfare: Education and looked-after children. *Child & Family Social Work,* 12(1), 1–10.

Berridge, D. 2012. Educating young people in care: What have we learned?. *Children and Youth Services Review,* 34(6), 1171–1175.

Berridge, D. 2017. The education of chidren in care: Agency and resilience. *Children and Youth Services Review,* 77, 86–93.

Berridge, S. & Brodie, I. 1998. *Children's Homes Revisited.* London: Jessica Kingsley Publishers.

Berridge, D., Dance, C., Beecham, J. & Field, S. 2008. *Educating Difficult Adolescents: Effective Education for Children in Public Care or with Emotional and Behavioural Difficulties.* London: Jessica Kingsley Publishers.

Biehal, N., Ellison, S. & Sinclair, I. 2009. *Characteristics, Outcomes and Meanings of Three Types of Permanent Placement – Adoption by Strangers, Adoption by*

Carers and Long-Term Foster Care. DCSF-RBX-09-11. London: Department for Children, Schools and Families (DCSF).

Biehal, N., Ellison, S., Baker, C. & Sinclair, I. 2010. *Belonging and Permanence: Outcomes in Long-Term Foster Care and Adoption.* London: British Association for Adoption and Fostering (BAAF).

Biehal, N., Sinclair, I. & Wade, J. 2015. Reunifying abused or neglected children: Decision-making and outcomes. *Child Abuse & Neglect,* 49, 107–118.

Billett, S., Thomas, S., Sim, C., Johnson, G., Hay, S. & Ryan, J. 2010. Constructing productive post-school transitions: An analysis of Australian schooling policies. *Journal of Education and Work,* 23(5), 471–489.

Blandon, J. & Gregg, P. 2004. Family income and educational attainment: A review of approaches and evidence for britain. *Oxford Review of Economic Policy,* 20(2), 245–263.

Blower, A., Addo, A., Hodgson, J., Lamington, L., & Towlson, K. 2004. Mental Health of 'Looked After' Children: A Needs Assessment. *Clinical Child Psychology and Psychiatry,* 9, 117.

Bluff, B., King, M. & McMahon, G. 2012. A phenomenological approach to care leavers' transition to higher education. *Procedia-Social and Behavioral Sciences,* 69, 952–959.

Boddy, J. 2011. The supportive relationship in 'public care': The relevance of social pedagogy. In: Cameron, C. & Moss, P. (eds.) *Social Pedagogy and Working with Children and Young People: Where Care and Education Meet.* London: Jessica Kingsley Publishers, 105–123.

Bon, C. 2009. Social pedagogy in France. In: Kornbeck, J. & Jensen, N. (eds.) *The Diversity of Social Pedagogy in Europe.* Bremen, Germany: Europaischer Hochschulverlag GmbH & Co., 34–45.

Bottrell, D. 2009. Understanding 'Marginal' Perspectives: Towards a Social Theory of Resilience. *Qualitative Social Work,* 8(3), 321–339.

Bowlby, J. 1969. *Attachment.* London: Penguin.

Bowlby, J. 1989. *A Secure Base: Clinical Applications of Attachment Theory.* London: Routledge.

Bovenschen, I., Lang, K., Zimmermann, J., Förthner, J., Nowacki, K., Roland, I. & Spangler, G. 2016. Foster children's attachment behavior and representation: Influence of children's pre-placement experiences and foster caregiver's sensitivity. *Child Abuse & Neglect,* 51, 323–335.

Braciszewski, J. & Stout, R. 2012. Substance use among current and former foster youth: A systematic review. *Children and Youth Services Review,* 34(12), 2337–2344.

Brandon, M., Belderson, P., Warren, C., Howe, D., Gardner, R., Dodsworth, J. & Black, J. 2008. *Analysing child deaths and serious injury through abuse and neglect: What can we learn? A biennial analysis of serious case reviews 2003–2005.* Research Report DCSF-RR023. Nottingham: Department for Children, Schools and Families.

Breen, R. 2010. Educational expansion and social mobility in the 20th century. *Social Forces,* 89(2), 365–388.

British Association of Social Workers. 2012. *Policy, Ethics and Human Rights Committee-Code of Ethics for Social Work: Statement of Principles.* Available at www.basw.co.uk/codeofethics/ (Accessed 19 May 2017).

Broadhurst, K., Grover, C. & Jamieson, J. 2009. Conclusion: Safeguarding children? In: Broadhurst, K., Grover, C. & Jamieson, J. (eds.) *Critical Perspectives on Safeguarding Children.* Chichester: Wiley-Blackwell, 247–258.

Brown, J. & Bednar, L. 2006. Foster parent perceptions of placement breakdown. *Children and Youth Services Review,* 28(12), 1497–1511.

Bryderup, I. & Trentel, M. 2013. The importance of social relationships for young people from a public care background. *European Journal of Social Work,* 16(1), 37–54.

Bullock, R., Courtney, M., Parker, R., Sinclair, I. & Thoburn, J. 2006. Can the corporate state parent? *Children and Youth Services Review,* 28(11), 1344–1358.

Bureau, J.-F., Easterbrooks, M. & Lyons-Ruth, K. 2009. Maternal depression symptoms in infancy: Unique contribution to children's depression sysmptoms in childhood and adolescence? *Development and Psychopathology,* 21(2), 519–537.

Buss, E. 2009. What the law should (and should not) learn from child development research. *Hofstra Law Review,* 38, 13–65.

Call, K. & Mortimer, J. 2001. *Arenas of Comfort in Adolescence: A Study of Adolescence in Context.* Mahwah, NJ: Lawrence Erlbaum Associates.

Calvert, M. 2009. From 'pastoral care' to 'care': Meanings and practices. *Pastoral Care in Education,* 27(4), 267–277.

Cameron, C. 2004. Social pedagogy and care: Danish and German pactice in young people's residential Care. *Journal of Social Work,* 4(2), 133–151.

Cameron, C. 2007. Education and self-reliance among care leavers. *Adoption & Fostering,* 31(1), 39–49.

Cameron, C., Jackson, J., Hauari, H. & Hollingworth, K. 2012. Continuing educational participation among children in care in five countries: Some issues of social class. *Journal of Education Policy,* 27(3), 387–399.

Cashmore, J. 2002. Promoting the participation of children and young people in care. *Child Abuse & Neglect,* 26, 837–847.

Centre for Social Justice. 2013. *'I Never Left Care, Care Left Me': Ensuring Good Corporate Parenting into Adulthood – A Briefing Paper for Peers on Proposed Amendments to the Children and Families Bill 2013.* London: Centre for Social Justice.

Centre for Social Justice. 2014. *Survivial of the Fittest? Improving Life Chances for Care Leavers.* London: Centre for Social Justice.

Centrepoint. 2010. *The Changing Face of Youth Homelessness: Trends in Homeless Young People's Support Needs.* London: Centrepoint.

Chaffin, M., Hanson, R., Saunders, B., Nichols, T., Barnett, D., Zeanah, C., Berliner, L., Egeland, B., Newman, E., Lyon, T., LeTourneau, E. & Miller-Perrin, C. 2006. Report of the APSAC task force on attachment therapy, reactive attachment disorder and attachment problems. *Child Maltreatment,* 11, 76–89.

Chartered Institute of Public Finance and Accountancy. 2011. *Smart Cuts? Public Spending on Children's Social Care: A Report Produced by the Chartered Institute of Public Finance and Accountancy for the National Society for the Prevention of Cruelty to Children (NSPCC).* London: NSPCC.

Chase, E., Simon, A. & Jackson, S. 2006. *In Care and After: A Positive Perspective.* London: Routledge.

Cheung, C., Lwin, K. & Jenkins, J. 2012. Helping youth in care succeed: Influence of caregiver involvement on academic achievement. *Children and Youth Services Review,* 34(6), 1092–1100.

Children's Bureau. 2015. *Adoption and Foster Care Analysis and Reporting System (AFCARS) FY 2014 Data. Preliminary Estimates for FY 2014 as of July 2015 No. 22.* U.S. Department of Health and Human Services, Administration for Children and Families, Administration on Children, Youth and Families.

Christiansen, Ø., Havik, T. & Anderssen, N. 2010. Arranging stability for children in long-term out-of-home care. *Children and Youth Services Review,* 32(7), 913–921.

Cicchetti, D. 2013. Annual research review: Resilient functioning in maltreated children – Past, present, and future perspectives. *Journal of Child Psychology and Psychiatry,* 54(4), 402–422.

Cicchetti, D., Rogosch, F. & Toth, S. 2006. Fostering secure attachment in infants in maltreating families through preventive interventions. *Development and Psychopathology,* 18(3), 623–649.

Clark, A. 2003. Unemployment as a social norm: Psychological evidence from panel data. *Journal of Labor Economics,* 21(2), 289–322.

Clark, A., Fritjers, P. & Shields, M. 2008. Relative income, happiness and utility: An explanation for the Easterlin paradox and other puzzles. *Journal of Economic Literature,* 46(1), 95–144.

Cohen, L., Tanis, T., Bhattacharjee, R., Nesci, C., Halmi, W. & Galynker, I. 2014. Are there differential relationships between different types of childhood maltreatment and different types of adult personality pathology? *Psychiatry Research,* 215, 192–201.

Coleman, J. 1974. *Relationships in adolescence.* London: Routledge and Keegan Paul.

Coleman, J. 2011. *The Nature of Adolescence,* 4th edition. London: Routledge.

Coleman, J. & Hagell, A. 2007. The nature of risk and resilience in adolescence. In J. Coleman, & A. Hagell, *Adolescent Risk and Resilience: Against the Odds.* Chichester: John Wiley and Sons, 1–16.

Coleman, K. & Wu, Q. 2016. Kinship care and service utilization: A review of predisposing, enabling, and need factors. *Children and Youth Services Review,* 61, 201–210.

Colton, M., Roberts, R. & Williams, M. 2008. The recruitment and retention of family foster-carers: An international and cross-cultural analysis. *British Journal of Social Work,* 38(5), 865–884.

Connelly, G. & Furnivall, J. 2013. Addressing low attainment of children in public care: The Scottish experience. *European Journal of Social Work,* 16(1), 88–104.

Courtney, J. & Prophet, R. 2011. Predictors of placement stability at the state level: The use of logistic regression to inform practice. *Child Welfare,* 90(2), 127–142.

Courtney, M., Dworsky, A., Ruth, G., Havlicek, J., Perez, A. & Keller, T. 2007. *Midwest Evaluation of the Adult Functioning of Former Foster Youth: Outcomes at Age 21.* Chicago, IL: Chapin Hall Center for Children.

Courtney, M., Dworsky, A., Brown, A., Cary, C., Love, K. & Vorhies, V. 2011. *Midwest Evaluation of the Adult Functioning of Former Foster Youth: Outcomes at Age 26.* Chicago, IL: Chaplin Hall.

Coussée, F., Bradt, L., Roose, R. & Bouverne-De Bie, M. 2010. The emerging social pedagogical paradigm in UK child and youth care: Deus Ex Machina or walking the beaten path? *British Journal of Social Work,* 40(3), 789–805.

Cree, V., Kay, H. & Tisdall, K. 2002. Research with children: Sharing the dilemmas. *Child & Family Social Work,* 7, 47–56.

Crittenden, P. 1988. Distorted patterns of relationship in maltreating families: The role of internal representation models. *Journal of Reproductive and Infant Psychology,* 6(3), 183–199.

Crittenden, P. 1992. Children's strategies for coping with adverse home environments: An interpretation using attachment theory. *Child Abuse and Neglect* 16, 329–343.

Crow, G., Wiles, R., Heath, S. & Charles, V. 2006. Research ethics and data quality: The implications of informed consent. *International Journal of Social Research Methodology,* 9(2), 83–95.

Cutuli, J., Goerge, R., Coulton, C., Schretzman, M., Crampton, D., Charvat, B., Lalich, M., Raithel, J., Gacitua, C. & Lee, E. 2016. From foster care to juvenile justice: Exploring characteristics of youth in three cities. *Children and Youth Services Review,* 67, 84–94.

Darmody, M., McMahon, L., Banks, J. & Gilligan, R. 2013. *Education of Children in Care in Ireland: An Exploratory Study.* Dublin: Ombudsman for Children.

Davison, M. & Burris, E. 2014. Transitioning foster care youth and their risk for homelessness: Policy, program, and budgeting shortcomings. *Human Welfare,* 3(1), 22–33.

Day, A., Dworsky, A., Fogarty, K. & Damashek, A. 2011. An examination of post-secondary retention and graduation among foster care youth enrolled in a four-year university. *Children and Youth Services Review,* 33(11), 2335–2341.

de Araujo, P. & Lagos, S. 2013. Self-esteem, education, and wages revisited. *Journal of Economic Psychology,* 34, 120–132.

del Valle, J., Lázaro-Visa, S., López, M. & Bravo, A. 2011. Leaving family care: Transitions to adulthood from kinship care. *Children and Youth Services Review,* 33(12), 2475–2481.

Department for Children, Schools and Families (DCSF). 2008. *Improving Behaviour and Attendance: Guidance on Exclusion from Schools and Pupil Referral Units.* London: Department for Children, Schools and Families (DCSF).

Department for Children, Schools and Families (DCSF). 2009. *The Role and Responsibilities of the Designated Teacher for Looked After Children: Statutory Guidance for School Governing Bodies. DCSF-01046–2009.* Nottingham: Department for Children, Schools and Families (DCSF).

Department for Children, Schools and Families (DCSF). 2010. *Promoting the Educational Achievement of Looked After Children: Statutory Guidance for Local Authorities, DCSF-00342–2010.* Nottingham: DCSF.

Department for Education (DfE). 2011. *A Child-Centred System: The Government's Response to the Munro Review of Child Protection.* London: Department for Education.

Department for Education (DfE). 2014. *Promoting the Education of Looked After Children: Statutory Guidance for Local Authorities. DFE-00520–2014.* London: Department for Education.

Department for Education (DfE). 2015. *The Children Act 1989 Guidance and Regulations Volume 2: Care Planning, Placement and Case Review.* London: Department for Education.

Department for Education (DfE). 2016. *Participation in Education, Training and Employment by 16–18 Year Olds in England: End 2015. SFR22/2016.* London: Department for Education/National Statistics.

Department for Education/National Statistics (DfE/NS). 2011. *Children Looked After in England (Including Adoption and Care Leavers) Year Ending 31 March 2011. SFR 21/2011.* London: Department for Education/National Statistics.

Department for Education/National Statistics (DfE/NS). 2013. *Children Looked After in England Including Adoption: 2012 to 2013. SFR36/2013.* London: Department for Education/National Statistics.

Department for Education/National Statistics (DfE/NS). 2016a. *Children Looked After in England Including Adoption: 2015 to 2016. SFR41/2016*. London: Department for Education/National Statistics.

Department for Education/National Statistics (DfE/NS). 2016b. *Outcomes for Children Looked After by Local Authorities in England, 31 March 2015. SFR 11/2016*. London: Department for Education/National Statistics.

Department for Education/National Statistics (DfE/NS). 2016c. *Participation Rates In Higher Education: Academic Years 2006/2007–2014/2015 (Provisional). SFR45/2016*. London: Department for Education/National Statistics.

Department for Education/National Statistics (DfE/NS), 2017. *Outcomes for Children Looked After by Local Authorities in England, 31 March 2016. SFR 12/2017*. London: Department for Education.

Deputy First Minister. 2017. *Ministerial Statement: Information Sharing Provisions in Relation to Part 4 & Part 5 of the Children and Young People (Scotland) Act 2014*. Available at: https://news.gov.scot/speeches-and-briefings/deputy-first-minister-ministerial-statement (Accessed 30 May 2017).

Dixon, J., Wade, J., Byford, S., Weatherly, H. & Lee, J. 2006. *Young People Leaving Care: A Study of Costs and Outcomes. Report to the DfES*. York: University of York, Social Work Research and Development Unit.

Dixon, R. & Nussbaum, M. 2012. Children's Rights and a capabilities approach: The question of special priority. Chicago Public law and legal theory working paper No. 384. *Cornell Law Review*, 97, 549–594.

Doyle Jr, J. 2013. Causal effects of foster care: An instrumental-variables approach. *Children and Youth Services Review*, 35(7), 1143–1151.

Drapeau, S., Saint-Jacques, M., Lepien, R., Begib, G. & Bernard, M. 2007. Processes that contribute to resilience among youth in foster care. *Journal of Adolescence*, 30, 977–999.

Driscoll, J. 2011. Making up lost ground: Challenges in supporting the educational attainment of looked after children beyond Key Stage 4. *Adoption and Fostering*, 35(2), 18–31.

Driscoll, J. 2013a. Supporting care leavers to fulfil their educational aspirations: Resilience, relationships and resistance to help. *Children and Society*, 27(2), 139–149.

Driscoll, J. 2013b. Supporting the educational transitions of looked after children at Key Stage 4: The role of virtual schools and designated teachers. *Journal of Children's Services*, 8(2), 110–122.

Dubois-Comtois, K., Bernier, A., Tarabulsy, G. M., Cyr, C.; St-Laurent, D., Lanctôt, A-S., St-Onge, J., Moss, E. & Béliveau, M-J. 2015. Behavior problems of children in foster care: Associations with foster mothers' representations, commitment, and the quality of mother–child interaction. *Child Abuse & Neglect*, 48, 119–130.

Dumont, M. & Provost, M. 1999. Resilience in adolescents: Protective role of social support, coping strategies, self-esteem, and social activities on experience of stress and depression. *Journal of Youth and Adolescence*, 28(3), 343–363.

Dunn, E., McLaughlin, K., Slopen, N., Rosand, J. & Smoller, J. 2013. Developmental timing of child maltreatment and symptoms of depression and suicidal ideation in young adulthood: Results from the national longitudinal study of adolescent health. *Depression and Anxiety*, 30(1), 955–964.

Easterbrooks, M. & Goldberg, W. 1990. Security of toddler-parent attachment: Relation to children's sociopersonality functioning during kindergarten. In: Greenberg, M., Cicchetti, D. & Cummings, M. (eds.) *Attachment in the Preschool Years: Theory, Research and Intervention.* Chicago, IL: University of Chicago Press, 221–244.

Easterlin, R., McVey, L., Switek, M., Sawangfa, O. & Smith Zweig, J. 2010. The happiness-income paradox revisted. *Proceedings of the National Academy of Sciences of the United States of America,* 107(52), 22463–22468.

Edinburgh Peace and Justice Centre. 2016. *Addressing the Needs of Unaccompanied Asylum Seeking Children and Child Refugees in Scotland.* Edinburgh: Edinburgh Peace and Justice Centre.

Eekelaar, J. 1986. The Emergence of Children's Rights. *Oxford Journal of Legal Studies,* 6(2), 161–182.

Eriksson, L. & Markström, A.-M. 2009. Social Pedagogy in a Swedish context. In: Kornbeck, J. & Jensen, N. (eds.) *The Diversity of Social Pedagogy in Europe.* Bremen, Germany: Europäischer Hochschulverlag GmbH & Co., 46–63.

Esping-Andersen, G. 1990. The three political economies of the welfare state. *International Journal of Sociology,* 20(3), 92–123.

European Commission. 2016. *EU Youth Report 2015: Joint Report of the Council and the Commission on the Implementation of the Renewed Framework for European Cooperation in the Youth Field (2010–2018).* Luxembourg: European Union.

Eurostat. 2016. *Unemployment Statistics: Data up to December 2016.* Available at: http://ec.europa.eu/eurostat/statistics-explained/index.php/Unemployment_statistics#Youth_unemployment_trends (Accessed 31 January 2017).

Evans, R., Brown, R., Rees, G. & Smith, P. 2017. Systematic review of educational interventions for looked-after children and young people: Recommendations for intervention development and evaluation. *British Educational Research Journal,* 43(1), 68–94.

Fagundes, C., Diamond, L. & Allen, K. 2012. Adolescent Attachment Insecurity and Parasympathetic Functioning Predict Future Loss Adjustment. *Personality and Social Psychology Bulletin,* 38(6), 821–832.

Fallesen, P. 2013. Time well spent: The duration of foster care and early adult labor market, educational, and health outcomes. *Journal of Adolescence,* 36(6), 1003–1011.

Family Justice Review Panel. 2011. *Family Justice Review – Interim Report.* London: Ministry of Jusice/Department for Education/Welsh Assembly Government.

Farmer, E. 2010. What factors relate to good placement outcomes in kinship care? *British Journal of Social Work,* 40(2), 426–444.

Farmer, E. & Moyers, S. 2008. *Kinship Care: Fostering Effective Family and Friends Placements.* London: Jessica Kingsley Publishers.

Farmer, E. & Lutman, E. 2010. What contributes to outcomes for neglected children who are reunified with their parents? Findings from a five-year follow-up study. *British Journal of Social Work,* 43(3), 559–578.

Fayle, J. 2011. *NAIRO Response to Family Justice Review Interim Report.* National Association of Independent Reviewing Officers (NAIRO).

Fearon, P., Shmueli-Goetz, Y., Viding, E., Fonagy, P. & Plomin, R. 2014. Genetic and environmental influences on adolescent attachment. *Journal of Child Psychology and Psychiatry,* 55(9), 1033–1041.

Ferguson, L. 2013. Not merely rights for children but children's rights: The theory gap and the assumption of the importance of children's rights. *International Journal of Children's Rights,* 21, 177–208.

Ferguson, H. & Wolkow, K. 2012. Educating children and youth in care: A review of barriers to school progress and strategies for change. *Children and Youth Services Review,* 34(6), 1143–1149.

Fergusson, D., McLeod, G. & Horwood, L. 2013. Childhood sexual abuse and adult developmental outcomes: Findings from a 30-year longitudinal study in New Zealand. *Child Abuse and Neglect,* 37(9), 664–674.

Fernandes-Alcantara, A. 2013. *Runaway and Homeless Youth: Demographics and Programs: CRS Report for Congress.* Washington, DC: Congressional Research Service.

Fineman, M. 2008. The vulnerable subject: Anchoring equality in the human condition. *Yale Journal of Law and Feminism,* 20(1), 1–23.

Finnie, R. 2012. Access to post-secondary education: The importance of culture. *Children and Youth Services Review* 34(6), 1161–1170.

Fionda, J. 2005. *Devils and Angels: Youth, Policy and Crime.* Oxford: Hart Publishing.

Fisher, P., Mannering, A., Van Scoyoc, A. & Graham, A. 2013. A translational neuroscience perspective on the importance of reducing placement instability among foster children. *Child Welfare,* 92(5), 9–36.

Fletcher-Campbell, F. 2008. Pupils who are "in care": What can schools do? In M. Baginsky (ed.), *Safeguarding Children and Schools.* London: Jessica Kingsley Publishers, 57–67.

Flynn, R. & Tessier, N. 2011. Promotive and risk factors as concurrent predictors of educational outcomes in supported transitional living: Extended care and maintenance in Ontario, Canada. *Children and Youth Services Review,* 33(12), 2498–2503.

Flynn, R., Marquis, R., Paquet, M.-P., Peeke, L. & Aubry, T. 2012. Effects of individual direct-instruction tutoring on foster children's academic skills: A randomized trial. *Children and Youth Services Review,* 34(6), 1183–1189.

Flynn, R., Tessier, N. & Coulombe, D. 2013. Placement, protective and risk factors in the educational success of young people in care: Cross-sectional and longitudinal analyses. *European Journal of Social Work,* 16(1), 70–87.

Foley, B. 2014. *Staying Power: Making the Raising of the Participation Age a Policy Success.* London: The Work Foundation (Lancaster University).

Font, S. 2014. Kinship and Nonrelative Foster Care: The Effect of Placement Type on Child Well-Being. *Child Development,* 85, 5, 2074–2090.

Font, S. 2015. Is higher placement stability in kinship foster care by virtue or design? *Child Abuse & Neglect,* 42, 99–111.

Font, S. & Maguire-Jack, K. 2013. Academic engagement and performance: Estimating the impact of out-of-home care for maltreated children. *Children and Youth Services Review,* 35(5), 856–864.

Ford, T., Vostanis, P., Meltzer, H. & Goodman, R. 2007. Psychiatric disorder among British children looked after by local authorities: Comparison with children living in private households. *British Journal of Psychiatry,* 190, 319–325.

Forrest, L., Hodgson, S., Parker, L. & Pearce, M. 2011. The influence of childhood IQ and education on social mobility in the Newcastle Thousand Families birth cohort. *BMC Public Health,* 11, 895–903.

Forsman, H. & Vinnerljung, B. 2012. Interventions aiming to improve school achievements of children in out-of-home care: A scoping review. *Children and Youth Services Review,* 34(6), 1084–1091.

Fortin, J. 2009. *Children's Rights and the Developing Law,* 3rd edition. Cambridge: Cambridge University Press.

Foster, E., Hillemeier, M. & Bai, Y. 2011. Explaining the disparity in placement instability among African-American and white children in child welfare: A Blinder–Oaxaca decomposition. *Children and Youth Services Review,* 33(1), 118–125.

Freeman, M. 1983. *The Rights and Wrongs of Children.* London: Francis Pinter.

Freeman, M. 1992. *The Moral Status of Children: Essays on the Rights of the Child.* The Hague: Martin Nijhoff Publishers.

Frost, N. & Stein, M. 1989. *The Politics of Child Welfare: Inequality, Power and Change.* Hemel Hempstead: Harvester Wheatsheaf.

Frydenberg, E. 2008. *Adolescent Coping: Advances in Theory, Research and Practice.* London: Routledge.

Furlong, A. 2009. Changing contexts, changing lives. In: Furlong, A. (ed.) *Handbook of Youth and Young Adulthood: New Perspectives and Agendas.* Oxford: Routledge, 1–2.

Gardiner, L. 2014. *Totalling the Hidden Talent: Youth Unemployment and Underemployment in England and Wales.* London: Local Government Association/Centre for Economic and Social Inclusion.

Gardner, R. & Brandon, M. 2008. Child protection: Crisis management or learning curve? *Public Policy Research,* 15(4), 177–186.

Gavin, H. 2011. Sticks and stones may break my bones: The effects of emotional abuse. *Journal of Aggression, Maltreatment & Trauma,* 20(5), 503–529.

Geenen, S. & Powers, L. 2007. "Tomorrow is another problem": The experiences of youth in foster care during their transition into adulthood. *Children and Youth Services Review,* 29(8), 1085–1101.

Gelhaar, T., Seiffge-Krenke, I., Borge, A., Cicognani, E., Cunha, M., Loncaric, D., Macek, P., Steinhausen, H.-C. & Winkler Metzke, C. 2007. Adolescent coping with everyday stressors: A seven-nation study of youth from central, eastern, southern, and northern Europe. *European Journal of Developmental Psychology,* 4(2), 129–156.

Gerber, A. 2007. Attachment, resilience, and psychoanalysis: Commentary on Hauser and Allen's "overcoming adversity in adolescence". *Psycholanalytic Inquiry,* 26(4), 585–594.

Gewirtz, S. 2002. *The Managerial School: Post-Welfarism and Social Justice in Education.* London: Routledge.

Gifford, E., Wells, R., Bai, Y., Troop, T., Miller, S. & Babinski, L. 2010. Pairing nurses and social workers in schools: North Carolina's school-based child and family support teams. *Journal of School Health,* 80(2), 104–107.

Gilbert, R., Kemp, A., Thoburn, J., Sidebotham, P., Radford, L, Glaser, D. & MacMillan, H. 2009a. Child maltreatment 2: Recognising and responding to child maltreatment. *Lancet,* 373, 167–180.

Gilbert, R., Spatz Widom, C., Browne, K., Fergusson, D., Webb, E. & Janson, S. 2009b. Child maltreatment 1: Burden and consequences of child maltreatment in high-income countries. *Lancet,* 373, 68–81.

Gilbert, N., Parton, N. & Skivenes, M. 2011. *Child Protection Systems: International Trends and Orientations.* New York: Oxford University Press.

Gillborn, D., & Youdell, D. (2000). *Rationing Education: Policy, practice, reform and equity.* Buckingham: Open University Press.

Gilligan, R. 2000. Adversity, resilience and young people: The protective value of positive school and spare time experiences. *Children and Society,* 14, 37–47.

Gilligan, R. 2008. Promoting resilience in young people in long term care-the relevance of roles and relationships in the domains of recreation and work. *Journal of Social Work Practice,* 22(1), 37–50.

Girtz, R. 2014. The mediation effect of education on self-esteem and wages. *Journal of Labour Research,* 35(4), 358–372.

Glaser, D. 2000. Child abuse and neglect and the brain – A review. *Journal of Child Psychology and Psychiatry,* 41(1), 97–116.

Goemans, A., van Geel, M. & Vedder, P. 2015. Over three decades of longitudinal research on the development of foster children: A meta-analysis. *Child Abuse & Neglect,* 42, 121–134.

Goldson, B. (2000). 'Children in need' or 'young offenders'? Hardening ideology, organizational change and new challenges for social work with children in trouble. *Child and Family Social Work,* (5): 255–265.

Goldson, B. 2002. New labour, social justice and children: Political calculation and the deserving-undeserving schism. *British Journal of Social Work,* 32(6), 683–695.

Goldson, B. & Muncie, J. 2006. *Youth Crime and Justice.* London: Sage.

Goldthorpe, J. 2016. Social class mobility in modern Britain: Changing structure, constant process. *Journal of the British Academy,* 4, 89–111.

Goodman, R. 2001. Psychometric properties of the Strengths and Difficulties Questionnaire (SDQ). *Journal of the American Academy of Child and Adolescent Psychiatry,* 40, 1337 1345.

Goodyear, A. 2013. Understanding looked-after childhoods. *Child and Family Social Work,* 18, 394–402.

Goossens, L. & Marcoen, A. 1999. Relationships during adolescence: Constructive vs.negative themes and relational dissatisfaction. *Journal of Adolescence,* 22, 65–79.

Graham, C. & Felton, A. 2006. Inequality and happiness: Insights from Latin America. *Journal of Economic Inequality,* 4, 107–122.

Greater London Authority Intelligence Unit, 2012. *2011 Census First Results: London Boroughs' Populations by Age and Sex.* London: Greater London Authority Intelligence Unit.

Greenberg, M., Speltz, M. & DeKlyen, M. 1993. The role of attachment in the early development of disruptive behavior problems. *Development and Psychopathology,* 5, 191–213.

Greger, H., Myhre, A., Lydersen, S. & Jozefiak, T. 2015. Previous maltreatment and present mental health in a high-risk adolescent population. *Child Abuse & Neglect,* 45, 122–134.

Greiff, S., Wüstenberg, S., Csapó, B., Demetriou, A., Hautamäki, A. & Martin, R. 2014. Domain-general problem solving skills and education in the 21st century. *Educational Research Review,* 13, 74–83.

Hagell, A. 2007. Anti-social behaviour. In J. Coleman & A. Hagell (eds), *Adolescent Risk and Resilience: Against the Odds.* Chichester: John Wiley and Sons, 125–142.

Hager, A. & Runtz, M. 2012. Physical and psychological maltreatment in childhood and later health problems in women: An exploratory investigation of the roles of perceived stress and coping strategies. *Child Abuse & Neglect,* 36(5), 393–403.

Hai, N. & Williams, A. 2004. *Implementing the Children (Leaving Care) Act 2000: The Experience of Eight London Boroughs.* London: National Children's Bureau.

Hämäläinen, J. 2015. Defining social pedagogy: Historical, theoretical and practical considerations. *British Journal of Social Work,* 45(3), 1022–1038.

Hannon, C., Bazalgette, L. & Wood, C. 2010. *In Loco Parentis.* London: Demos.

Hansbauer, P. 2008. Structural dynamics in society and innovations in the German residential care system. In: Peters, F. (ed.) *Residential Child Care and Its Alternatives: International Perspectives.* Stoke on Trent: Trentham Books Limited, 51–70.

Harker, R., Dobel-Ober, D., Berridge, D. & Sinclair, R. 2004. *Taking Care of Education: An Evaluation of the Education of Looked after Children.* London: National Children's Bureau.

Harkin, C. & Houston, N. 2016. Reviewing the literature on the breakdown of foster care placements for young people: Complexity and the social work task. *Child Care in Practice,* 22(2), 98–112.

Harper, J. & Schmidt, F. 2012. Preliminary effects of a group-based tutoring program for children in long-term foster care. *Children and Youth Services Review,* 34(6), 1176–1182.

Harris, S., Jackson, L., O'Brien, K. & Pecora, P. 2010. Ethnic group comparisons in mental health outcomes of adult alumni of foster care. *Children and Youth Services Review,* 32(2), 171–177.

Hart, D. & Williams, A. 2013. *Putting Corporate Parenting into Practice,* 2nd edition. London: National Children's Bureau.

Harter, S. 2012. *The Construction of the Self.* New York: The Guildford Press.

Harvey, A., McNamara, P. & Andrewartha, L. 2016. Towards a national policy framework for care leavers in Australian higher education. In: Mendes, P. & Snow, P. (eds). *Young People Transitioning from Out-of-Home Care: International Research, Policy and Practice.* London: Palgrave Macmillan, 93–113.

Healy, K. & Oltedal, S., 2010. An institutional comparison of child protection systems in Australia and Norway focused on workforce retention. *Journal of Social Policy,* 39(2), 255–274.

Heath, S., Charles, V., Crow, G. & Wiles, R. 2007. Informed consent, gatekeepers and go-betweens: Negotiating consent in child-and youth-oriented institutions. *British Educational Research Journal,* 33(3), 403–417.

Heinz, W. 2009. Youth transitions in and age of uncertainty. In: Furlong, A. (ed.) *Handbook of Youth and Young Adultood: New Perspectives and Agendas.* Oxford: Routledge, 3–13.

Herrick, M. & Piccus, W. 2005. Sibling connections: The importance of nurturing sibling bonds in the foster care system. *Children and Youth Services Review,* 27(7), 845–861.

Hershenberg, R., Davila, J., Yoneda, A., Starr, L., Miller, M., Stroud, C. & Feinstein, B. 2011. What I like about you: The association between adolescent attachment security and emotional behavior in a relationship promoting context. *Journal of Adolescence,* 34(5), 1017–1024.

Hessle, S. 2013. Sweden. In: Welbourne, P. & Dixon, J. (eds.) *Child Protection and Child Welfare: A Global Appraisal of Cultures, Policy and Practice.* London: Jessica Kingsley Publishers, 25–44.

HM Government. 2015. *Working Together to Safeguard Children: A Guide to Inter-Agency Working to Safegurd and Promote the Welfare of Children.* London: HM Government.

Hocking, E., Simons, R. & Surette, R. 2016. Attachment style as a mediator between childhood maltreatment and the experience of betrayal trauma as an adult. *Child Abuse & Neglect, 52,* 94–101.

Hodgen, J., Marks, R. & Pepper, D. 2013. *Towards Universal Participation in Post-16 Mathematics: Lessons from High-Performing Countries.* London: Nuffield Foundation.

Höjer, I., Johansson, H., Cameron, C. & Jackson, J. 2008. *State of the Art Consolidated Literature Review: The Educational Pathways of Young People from a Public Care Background in Five EU countries.* YIPPEE *Young People from a Public Care Background: Establishing a Baseline of Attainment and Progression beyond Compulsory Schooling in Five EU countries.* Thomas Coram Research Unit. London: Institute of Education, University of London.

Höjer, I. & Johansson, H. 2013. School as an opportunity and resilience factor for young people placed in care. *European Journal of Social Work,* 16(1), 22–36.

Holland, S. 2009. Listening to children in care: A review of methodological and theoretical approaches to understanding looked after children's perspectives. *Children & Society,* 23(3), 226–235.

Holmes, E., Miscampbell, G. & Robin, B. 2013. *Reforming Social Work: Improving Social Worker Recruitment, Training and Retention.* London: Policy Exchange.

Holtan, A., Handegård, B., Thørnblad, R. & Vis, S. 2013. Placement disruption in long-term kinship and nonkinship foster care. *Children and Youth Services Review,* 35(7), 1087–1094.

Hollingsworth, K. 2013a. Securing responsibilty, achieving parity? The legal support for children leaving custody. *Legal Studies,* 33(1), 22–45.

Hollingsworth, K. 2013b. Theorising children's rights in youth justice: The significance of autonomy and foundational rights. *The Modern Law Review,* 76(6), 1046–1069.

Hollingsworth, K. & Jackson, S. 2016. Falling off the ladder: Using focal theory to understand and improve the educational experiences of young people in transition from public care. *Journal of Adolescence,* 52, 146–153.

Honey, K., Rees, P. & Griffey, S. 2011. Investigating self-perceptions and resilience in looked after children. *Educational Psychology in Practice,* 27(1), 37–52.

Hook, J. & Courtney, M. 2011. Employment outcomes of former foster youth as young adults: The importance of human, personal, and social capital. *Children and Youth Services Review,* 33(10), 1855–1865.

House of Commons Children, Schools and Families Committee (HC CSFC). 2009. *Looked after Children: Third Report of Session 2008–09, Volume I Report, Together with Formal Minutes. HC111-I.* London: The Stationery Office.

House of Commons Education Committee. 2014. *Into Independence, Not Out of Care, 16 Plus Care Options. Second Report of Session 2014–15. HC259.* London: The Stationery Office Limited.

Hyde, J. & Kammerer, N. 2009. Adolescents' perspectives on placement moves and congregate settings: Complex and cumulative instabilities in out-of-home care. *Children and Youth Services Review,* 31(2), 265–273.

IOM (Institute of Medicine) and NRC (National Research Council). 2014. *New Directions in Child Abuse and Neglect Research.* Washington, DC: The National Academies Press.

Jackson, S. 2007. Care leavers, exclusion and access to higher education. In: Abrams, D., Christian, J. & Gordon, D. (eds.) *Multidisciplinary Handbook of Social Exclusion Research.* Hoboken, NJ: John Wiley and Sons Ltd, 115–135.

Jackson, S. 2010. Reconnecting care and education: From the Children Act 1989 to Care Matters. *Journal of Children's Services,* 5(3), 48–59.

Jackson, S. 2013a. Introduction. In: Jackson, S. (ed.) *Pathways through Education for Young People in Care: Ideas from Research and Practice.* London: BAAF, 1–8.

Jackson, S. 2013b. Reconnecting care and education: From the Children Act 1999 to Care Matters. In S. Jackson, *Pathways through Education for Young People in Care.* London: British Association for Adoption and Fostering, 11–26.

Jackson, S. & Ajayi, S. 2007. Foster care and higher education. *Adoption and Fostering,* 31(1), 62–72.

Jackson, S., Ajayi, S. & Quigley, M. 2003. *By Degrees: The First Year, from Care to University.* London: The Frank Buttle Trust.

Jackson, S., Ajayi, S. & Quigley, M. 2005. *Going to University from Care: Final Report of the By Degrees Project.* London: Institute of Education.

Jackson, S. & Cameron, C. 2010. *Young People from a Public Care Background: Establishing a Baseline of Attainment and Progression beyond Compulsory Schooling in Five EU Countries.* London: Institute of Education, University of London.

Jackson, S. & Cameron, C. 2011. *Final Report of the YiPPEE Project-WP12: Young People from a Public Care Background: Pathways to Further and Higher Education in Five European Countries.* Thomas Coram Research Unit. London: Institute of Education.

Jackson, S. & Cameron, C. 2012. Leaving care: Looking ahead and aiming higher. *Children and Youth Services Review,* 34(6), 1107–1114.

Jackson, S. & Martin, P. 1998. Surviving the care system: Education and resilience. *Journal of Adolescence,* 21(5), 569–583.

Jackson, Y., Gabrielli, J., Fleming, K., Tunno, A. & Makanui, P. 2014. Untangling the relative contribution of maltreatment severity and frequency to type of behavioral outcome in foster youth. *Child Abuse & Neglect,* 38(7), 1147–1159.

Janer, A. & Úcar, X. 2017. Analysing the dimensions of social pedagogy from an international perspective. *European Journal of Social Work,* 20(2), 203–218.

Jelicic, H., La Valle, I. & Hart, D. 2014. *The role of Independent Reviewing Officers (IROs) in England.* London: National Children's Bureau.

Johansson, H. & Höjer, I. 2012. Education for disadvantaged groups – Structural and individual challenges. *Children and Youth Services Review,* 34(6), 1135–1142.

Johnson, W., Brett, C. & Deary, I. 2010. The pivotal role of education in the association between ability and social class attainment: A look across three generations. *Intelligence,* 38, 55–65.

Joseph, M., O'Connor, T., Briskman, J., Maughan, B. & Scott, S. 2014. The formation of secure new attachments by children who were maltreated: An observational study of adolescents in foster care. *Development and Psychopathology,* 26, 67–80.

Joubert, D., Webster, L. & Hackett, R. 2012. Unresolved attachment status and trauma-related symptomatology in maltreated adolescents: An examination of cognitive mediators. *Child Psychiatry & Human Development,* 43, 471–483.

Katz, I. & Hetherington, R., 2006. Co-operating and communicating: A European perspective on integrating services for children. *Child Abuse Review,* 15(6), 429–439.

Kay, C. & Green, J. 2013. Reactive attachment disorder following early maltreatment: Systematic evidence beyond the institution. *Journal of Abnormal Child Psychology,* 41, 571–581.

Kelly, B., McShane, T., Davidson, G., Pinkerton, G., Gilligan, E. & Webb, P. 2016. *You Only Leave Once? Transitions and Outcomes for Care Leavers with Mental Health and/or Intellectual Disabilities: Final report.* Belfast: QUB.

Kemp, R. 2011. Social pedagogy: Differences and links to existing child care practice. *Children Australia,* 36(4), 199–206.

Kemp, R. 2015. Treasuring the Social in Social Pedagogy Children Australia 40(4), 348–350.

Kennedy, E. 2013. *Children and Young People in Custody 2012–13: An Analysis of 15–18-year-olds' Perceptions of Their Experiences in Young Offender Institutions.* Norwich: HM Inspectorate of Prisons/Youth Justice Board.

Khoo, E. & Skoog, V. 2014. The road to placement breakdown: Foster parents' experiences of the events surrounding the unexpected ending of a child's placement in their care. *Qualitative Social Work,* 13(2), 255–269.

Khoo, E., Skoog, V. & Dalin, R. 2012. In and out of care. A profile and analysis of children in the out-of-home care system in Sweden. *Children and Youth Services Review,* 34(5), 900–907.

Kirby, P. 2006. *Vulnerability and Violence: The Impact of Globalisation.* London: Pluto Press.

Kirk, C., Lewis, R., Brown, K., Nilsen, C. & Colvin, D. 2012. The gender gap in educational expectations among youth in the foster care system. *Children and Youth Services Review,* 34(9), 1683–1688.

Kloep, M. 1999. Love is all you need? Focusing on adolescents' life concerns from an ecological point of view. *Journal of Adolescence,* 22(1), 49–63.

Kobolt, A. & Dekleva, B. 2008. The professionalism of child and youth care practice: Professionalising social pedagogy-from practice to theory and back to practice. In: Peters, F. (ed.) *Residential Child Care and Its Alternatives: International Perspectives.* Stoke on Trent: Trentham Books Limited, 79–97.

Kornbeck, J. & Jensen, N. 2009. Introduction: Social pedagogy in Europe – diverse with common features. In: Kornbeck, J. & Jensen, N. R. (eds.) *The Diversity of Social Pedagogy in Europe.* Bremen: Europäischer Hochschulverlag GmbH & Co., 1–10.

Lee, J.-S. 2014. The attainability of university degrees and their labour market benefits for young Australians. *Higher Education,* 68(3), 449–469.

Lee, C. & Berrick, J. 2014. Experiences of youth who transition to adulthood out of care: Developing a theoretical framework. *Children and Youth Services Review,* 46, 78–84.

Leeson, C. 2007. My life in care: Experiences of nonparticipation in decision-making processes. *Child & Family Social Work,* 12(3), 268–277.

Limke, A., Showers, C. & Zeigler-Hill, V. 2010. Emotional and sexual maltreatment: Anxious attachment mediates psychological adjustment. *Journal of Social and Clinical Psychology,* 29(3), 347–367.

Lobbestael, J., Arntz, A. & Bernstein, D. 2010. Disentangling the relationship between different types of childhood maltreatment and personality disorders. *Journal of Personality Disorders,* 24(3), 285–295.

Lonne, B., Parton, N., Thomson, J. & Harries, M. 2009. *Reforming Child Protection.* Abingdon: Routledge.

Lonne, B., Harries, M. & Lantz, S. 2013. Workforce development: A pathway to reforming child protection systems in Australia. *British Journal of Social Work,* 43(8), 1630–1648.

Lowell, A., Renk, K. & Adgate, A. 2014. The role of attachment in the relationship between childmaltreatment and later emotional and behavioral functioning. *Child Abuse & Neglect,* 38(9), 1436–1449.

Luthar, S. & Cicchetti, D. 2000. The concept of resilience: Implications for interventions and social policies. *Development and Psychopathology,* 12(4), 857–885.

Lutman, E., Hunt, J. & Waterhouse, S. 2009. Placement stability for children in kinship care: A long-term follow-up of children placed in kinship care through care proceedings. *Adoption & Fostering,* 33(3), 28–39.

Maclean, M., Sims, S., O'Donnell, M. & Gilbert, R. 2016. Out-of-home care versus in-home care for children who have been maltreated: A systematic review of health and wellbeing outcomes. *Child Abuse Review,* 25(4), 251–272.

MacDonald, R. 2007. Social exclusion, risk and young adulthood. In Coleman, J. & Hagell A. (Eds.), *Adolescent Risk and Resilience: Against the Odds.* Chichester: John Wiley and Sons, 143–164.

Main, M. & Solomon, J. 1990. Procedures for identifying infants as disorganized/disoriented during the ainsworth strange situation test. In: Greenberg, M., Cicchetti, D. & Cummings, E. (eds.) *Attachment in the Preschool Years: Theory, Research and Intervention.* Chicago, IL: University of Chicago Press, 121–160.

Mallon, J. 2007. Returning to education after care: Protective factors in the development of resilience. *Adoption and Fostering,* 31(1), 106–116.

Malvaso, C., Delfabbro, P. & Day, A. 2017. The child protection and juvenile justice nexus in Australia: A longitudinal examination of the relationship between maltreatment and offending. *Child Abuse & Neglect,* 64, 32–46.

Mann, A., Massey, D., Glover, P., Kashefpadkel, E. & Dawkins, J. 2013. *Nothing in Common: The Career Aspirations of Young Britons Mapped against Projected Labour Market Demand (2010–2020).* London: Education and Employers Taskforce/UK Commission for Employment and Skills.

Mannay, D., Staples, E., Hallett, S., Roberts, L., Rees, A., Evans, R. & Andrews, D. 2015. *Understanding the Educational Experiences and Opinions, Attainment, Achievement and Aspirations of Looked after Children in Wales. Social Research Number 62/2015.* Cardiff: Welsh Government.

Martin, P. & Jackson, S. 2002. Educational success for children in public care: Advice from a group of high achievers. *Child & Family Social Work,* 7(2), 121–130.

Masson, J. 2000. Researching children's perspectives: Legal issues. In: Lewis, A. & Lindsay, G. (eds.) *Researching Children's Perspectives.* Buckingham and Philadelphia, PA: Open University Press, 34–45.

Masten, A., Best, K. & Garmezy, N. 1990. Resilience and development: Contributions from the study of children who overcome adversity. *Development and Psychopathology,* 2, 425–444.

Masten, A., Burt, K., Roisman, G., Obradovic, J., Long, J. & Tellegen, A. 2004. Resources and resilience in the transition to adulthood: Continuity and change. *Development and Psychopathology,* 16, 1071–1094.

McBeath, B., Kothari, B., Blakeslee, J., Lamson-Siu, E., Bank, L., Linares, L., Waid, J., Sorenson, P., Jimenez, J., Pearson, E. & Shlonsky, A. 2014. Intervening to improve outcomes for siblings in foster care: Conceptual, substantive, and methodological dimensions of a prevention science framework. *Children and Youth Services Review,* 39, 1–10.

McClung, M. & Gayle, V. 2010. Exploring the care effects of multiple factors on educational achievement of children looked after at home and away from home: An investigation of two Scottish local authorities. *Child and Family Social Work,* 15, 409–431.

McCoy, H., Curtis McMillen, J. & Spitznagel, E. 2008. Older youth leaving the foster care system: Who, what, when, where, and why? *Children and Youth Services Review,* 30(7), 735–745.

McFadden, P., Campbell, A. & Taylor, B. 2015. Resilience and burnout in child protection social work: Individual and organisational themes from a systematic literature review. *British Journal of Social Work,* 45(5), 1546–1563.

McGloin, J. & Widom, C. 2001. Resilience among abused and neglected children grown up. *Development and Psychopathology,* 13, 1021–1038.

McLean, C., Rosenbach, S., Capaldi, S. & Foa, E. 2013. Social and academic functioning in adolescents with child sexual abuse-related PTSD. *Child Abuse and Neglect,* 37(9), 675–678.

McLeod, A. 2010. 'A friend and an equal': Do young people in care seek the impossible from their social workers? *British Journal of Social Work,* 40, 772–788.

Meschi, E., Vignoles, A. & Cassen, R. 2014. Post-secondary school type and academic achievement. *The Manchester School,* 82 (2), 183–201.

Michalos, A. 2008. Education, happiness and wellbeing. *Social Indicators Research,* 87, 347–366.

MindFull. 2013. *"Alone with My thoughts": Recommendations for a New Approach to Young People's Mental Health Support.* MindFull.

Minow, M. 1986. Rights for the next generation: A feminist approach to children's rights. *Harvard Women's Law Journal,* 9, 1–24.

Monserrat, C., Casas, F. & Malo, S. 2013. Delayed educational pathways and risk of social exclusion: The case of young people from public care in Spain. *European Journal of Social Work,* 16(1), 6–21.

Mooney, M., Statham, J., Monck, M. & Chambers, H. 2009. *Promoting the health of looked after children, a study to inform revision of the 2000 guidance DCSF-RR125.* London: Department for Children, Schools and Families.

Moran, P., Coffey, C., Romaniuk, H., Olsson, C., Borschmann, R., Carlin, J. & Patton, G. 2012. The natural history of self-harm from adolescence to young adulthood: A population-based cohort study. *Lancet,* 379, 236–243.

Morgan, R. 2014. *The Children's Views Digest.* Manchester: Ofsted.

Moss, E. & St-Laurent, D. 2001. Attachment at school age and academic performance. *Developmental Psychology,* 37, 863–874.

Moss, P. & Cameron, C. 2011. Social pedagogy: Future directions?. In: Moss, P. & Cameron, C. (eds.) *Social Pedagogy and Working with Children and Young People: Where Care and Education Meet.* London: Jessica Kingsley Publishers, 195–209.

Muller, R. T., Thornback, K. & Bedi, R. 2012. Attachment as a mediator between childhood maltreatment and adult symptomatology. *Journal of Family Violence,* 27, 243–255.

Munro, E. 2011. *The Munro Review of Child Protection: Final Report – A Child-Centred System.* London: The Stationery Office.

Munro, E., Lushey, C., National Care Advisory Service, Maskell-Graham, D. & Ward, H. with Holmes, L. 2012. *Evaluation of the Staying Put: 18+ Family Placement*

Pilot Programme: Final Report. DfE RR-191. Loughborough: Loughborough University.

Murphy, A., Steele, M., Dube, S., Bate, J., Bonuck, K., Meissner, P., Goldman, H. & Steele, H. 2014. Adverse Childhood Experiences (ACEs) Questionnaire and Adult Attachment Interview (AAI): Implications for parent child relationships. *Child Abuse & Neglect,* 38, 224–233.

Murray, C. 2005. Children and young people's participation and non-participation in research. *Adoption and Fostering,* 29(1), 57–66.

Myers, J. 2008. A short history of child protection in America. *Family Law Quarterly,* 42(3), 449–463.

Nandy, S. & Selwyn, J. 2012. Kinship care and poverty: Using census data to examine the extent and nature of kinship care in the UK. *British Journal of Social Work,* 43(8), 1649–1666.

National Collaborating Centre for Mental Health (NCCMH). 2015. *Children's Attachment: Attachment in Children and Young People Who Are Adopted from Care, in Care or at High Risk of Going into Care. NICE Guideline 26: Methods, Evidence and Recommendations.* Leicester: The British Psychological Society & The Royal College of Psychiatrists.

National Institute of Adult Continuing Education (England and Wales) (NIACE). 2015. *Supporting Care Leavers in Further Education: A Guide to Good Practice in Colleges Achieving the Buttle UK Quality Mark.* Leicester: NIACE.

Noonan, K., Matone, M., Zlotnik, S., Hernandez-Mekonnen, R., Watts, C., Rubin, D. & Mollen, C. 2012. Cross-system barriers to educational success for children in foster care: The front line perspective. *Children and Youth Services Review,* 34(2), 403–408.

Norgate, R. 2012. Social workers' perspectives on the placement instability of looked after children. *Adoption and Fostering,* 36(2), 4–18.

Nussbaum, M. 2000. *Women and Human Development: The Capabilities Approach.* Cambridge: Cambridge University Press.

Nussbaum, M. 2003. Capabilities as fundamental entitlements: Sen and social justice. *Feminist Economics,* 9(2–3), 33–59.

Nussbaum, M. 2011. *Creating Capabilities: The Human Development Approach.* Cambridge, MA: Harvard University Press.

O'Brien, M. 2012. Knowledge transfer resulting from the Improving Educational Outcomes for Children in Care conference: How it is helping a child welfare organization to build a long term educational strategy. *Children and Youth Services Review,* 34(6), 1150–1153.

Obsuth, I., Hennighausen, K., Brumariu, L. & Lyons-Ruth, K. 2014. Disorganized behavior in adolescent-parent interaction: Relations to attachment state of mind, partner abuse, and psychopathology. *Child Development,* 85, 370–387.

OECD, 2014. *The OECD Innovation Strategy: Getting a Head Start on Tomorrow.* Paris: OECD Publishing.

OECD, 2015. *Education at a Glance 2015: OECD Indicators.* Paris: OECD Publishing.

Ofsted, 2008. *Safeguarding Children: The Third Joint Chief Inspectors' Report on Arrangements to Safeguard Children.* London: Ofsted.

Ofsted. 2011. *The Annual Report of her Majesty's Chief Inspector of Education, Children's Services, and Skills 2010/11.* London: Ofsted.

Ofsted. 2012. *The Impact of Virtual Schools on the Educational Progress of Looked after Children.* London: Ofsted.

Ofsted. 2013a. *2012/13 Social Care.* London: Ofsted.

Ofsted. 2013b. *Independent Reviewing Officers: Taking Up the Challenge?* London: Ofsted.

Ofsted. 2014. *From a Distance: Looked after Children Living Away from Their Home Area.* London: Ofsted.

O'Higgins, A., Sebba, J. & Luke, N. 2015. *What is the Relationship between Being in Care and the Educational Outcomes of Children? An International Systematic Review.* University of Oxford, The Rees Centre. Oxford: University of Oxford.

Okpych, N. 2012. Policy framework supporting youth aging-out of foster care through college: Review and recommendations. *Children and Youth Services Review,* 34(7), 1390–1396.

Okpych, N. & Courtney, M. 2014. Does education pay for youth formerly in foster care? Comparison of employment outcomes with a national sample. *Children and Youth Services Review,* 43, 18–28.

Olsson, M., Egelund, T. & Høst, A. 2012. Breakdown of teenage placements in Danish out-of-home care. *Child & Family Social Work* 17, 13–22.

Oosterman, M., Schuengel, C., Slot, N., Bullens, R. & Doreleijers, T. 2007. Disruptions in foster care: A review and meta-analysis. *Children and Youth Services Review,* 29(1), 53–76.

Oshri, A., Sutton, T., Clay-Warner, J. & Miller, J. 2015. Child maltreatment types and risk behaviors: Associations with attachment style and emotion regulation dimensions. *Personality and Individual Differences,* 73, 127–133.

O'Sullivan, A., Westerman, R., McNamara, P. & Mains, A. 2013. Closing the gap: Investigating the barriers to educational achievement for looked after children. In: Jackson, S. (ed.) *Pathways through Education for Young People in Care: Ideas from Research and Practice.* London: British Association for Adoption and Fostering, 66–77.

Osuwu-Bempah, K. 2010. *The Well-Being of Children in Care: A New Approach for Improving Developmental Outcomes.* Abingdon: Routledge.

Owen, C. & Statham, J. 2009. *Disproportionality in Child Welfare-Prevalence of Black and Ethnic Minority Children within 'Looked After' and 'Children in Need' Populations and on Child Protection Registers in England (No. DCSF-RR-124).* London: DCSF.

Pascuzzo, K., Cyr, C. & Moss, E. 2013. Longitudinal association between adolescent attachment, adult romantic attachment, and emotion regulation strategies. *Attachment & Human Development,* 15(1), 83–103.

Pears, K., Kim, H., Buchanan, R. & Fisher, P. 2015. Adverse consequences of school mobility for children in foster care: A prospective longitudinal study. *Child Development,* 86(4), 1210–1226.

Pecora, P. 2012. Maximizing educational achievement of youth in foster care and alumni: Factors associated with success. *Children and Youth Services Review,* 34(6), 1121–1129.

Pecora, P., Kessler, R., O'Brien, K., White, C., Williams, J., Hiripi, E., English, D., White, J. & Herrick, M. 2006. Educational and employment outcomes of adults formerly placed in foster care: Results from the Northwest foster care alumni study. *Children and Youth Services Review,* 28(12), 1459–1481.

Peter, C., Dworsky, A., Courtney, M. & Pollack, H. 2009. *Extending Foster Care to Age 21: Weighing the Costs to Government against the Benefits to Youth.* Chicago, IL: Chapin Hall at the University of Chicago.

Petersen, A., Joseph, J. & Feit, M. (eds.). 2014. *New Directions in Child Abuse and Neglect Research.* Washington, DC: National Academies Press (US).

Petrie, P. 2013. Social Pedagogy in the UK: Gaining a firm foothold? *Education Policy Analysis Archives,* 21(37), 1–16.

Petrie, P. & Simon, A. 2006. Residential care: Lessons from Europe. In: Chase, E., Simon, A. & Jackson, S. *In care and after: A positive perspective.* London: Routledge, 115–136.

Petrie, P. & Cameron, C. 2009. Importing social pedagogy? In: Kornbeck, J. & Jensen, N. (eds.) *The Diversity of Social Pedagogy in Europe.* Bremen: Europäischer Hochschulverlag GmbH & Co., 145–168.

Pinkerton, J. 2011. Contructing a global understanding of the social ecology of leaving out of home care. *Children and Youth Services Review,* 33(12), 2412–2416.

Pösö, T., Skivenes, M. & Hestbæk, A.-D. 2014. Child protection systems within the Danish, Finnish and Norwegian welfare states – Time for a child centric approach? *European Journal of Social Work,* 17(4), 475–490.

Power, S. 1996. *The Pastoral and the Academic: Conflict and Contradiction in the Curriculum.* London: Cassell.

Poyser, M. 2013. Is inclusion always best for young people in care? A view from the classroom. In S. Jackson (ed.). *Pathways through Education for Young People in Care: Ideas from Research and Practice.* London: British Association for Adoptions and Fostering (BAAF), 129–134.

Prior, V. & Glaser, D. 2006. *Understanding Attachment and Attachment Disorders: Theory, Evidence and Parctice.* London: Jessica Kingsley Pubishers.

Pryce, J., Napolitano, L. & Samuels, G. 2017. Transition to adulthood of former foster youth: Multilevel challenges to the help-seeking process. *Emerging Adulthood,* 1–11.

Pullmann, H. & Allik, J. 2008. Relations of academic and general self-esteem to school achievement. *Personality and Individual Differences,* 45, 559–564.

Putnam, R. 2015. *Our Kids: The American Dream in Crisis.* New York: Simon & Schuster.

Rácz, A. & Korintus, M. 2013. Enabling young people with a care background to stay in education in Hungary: Accommodation with conditions and support. *European Journal of Social Work,* 16(1), 55–69.

Randle, M., Ernst, D., Leisch, F. & Dolnicar, S. 2017. What makes foster carers think about quitting? Recommendations for improved retention of foster carers. *Child & Family Social Work,* 22(3), 1175–1186.

Rawson, A. 2016. *The Caring University in 2016: Practice, Partnership and Strategy with the Care Experienced Student.* London: Buttle UK/Action on Access.

Reeve, K. & Batty, E. 2011. *The Hidden Truth about Homelessness.* London: Crisis.

Rholes, W., Paetzold, R. & Kohn, J. 2016. Disorganized attachment mediates the link from early trauma to externalizing behavior in adult relationships. *Personality and Individual Differences,* 90, 61–65.

Rock, S., Michelson, D., Thomson, S. & Day, C. 2015. Understanding foster placement instability for looked after children: A systematic review and narrative synthesis of quantitative and qualitative evidence. *British Journal of Social Work,* 45(1), 177–203.

Romano, E., Babchishin, L., Marquis, R. & Fréchette, S. 2015. Childhood maltreatment and educational outcomes. *Trauma, Violence & Abuse,* 16(4), 418–437.

Rutter, M. 1985. Resilience in the face of adversity: Protective factors and resistance to psychiatric disorders. *British Journal of Psychiatry*, 147, 589–611.

Rutter, M. 2000. Children in substitute care: Some conceptual considerations and research implications. *Children and Youth Services Review*, 22(9/10), 685–703.

Rutter, M. 2006. Implications of resilience concepts for scientific understanding. In Lester, B., Masten, M. & McEwen, B. *Resilience in Children: Annals of the New York academy of sciences*, Vol. 1094. Boston, MA: Blackwell Publishing, 1–12.

Sameroff, A., Gutman, L., & Peck, S. 2003. Adaptation among youth facing multiple risks. In S. Luthar (ed.), *Resilience and Vulnerability*. Cambridge: Cambridge University Press, 364–391.

Samuels, G. & Pryce, J. 2008. "What doesn't kill you makes you stronger": Survivalist self-reliance as resilience and risk among young adults aging out of foster care. *Children and Youth Services Review*, 30(10), 1198–1210.

Savage, J. 2014. The association between attachment, parental bonds and physically aggressive and violent behavior: A comprehensive review. *Aggression and Violent Behavior*, 19, 164–178.

Scherger, S. & Savage, M. 2010. Cultural transmission, educational attainment and social mobility. *The Sociological Review*, 58(3), 406–428.

Schofield, G. 2001. Resilience and family placement: A lifespan perspective. *Adoption and Fostering*, 25(3), 6–19.

Scruggs, L. & Allan, J. 2008. Social stratification and welfare regimes for the twenty-first century: Revisiting the three worlds of welfare capitalism. *World Policy*, 60(4), 642–664.

Sebba, J., Berridge, D., Luke, N., Fletcher, J., Bell, K., Strand, S., Thomas, S., Sinclair, I. & O'Higgins, A. 2015. *The Educational Progress of Looked After Children in England – Linking Care and Educational Data*. Oxford: University of Oxford, Rees Centre.

Seiffge-Krenke, I. 1995. *Stress, Coping, and Relationships in Adolescence*. Mahwah, NJ: Lawrence Erlbaum Associates, Inc.

Sen, A. 1979. *Equality of What? The Tanner Lecture on Human Values*. Stanford, CA: Stanford University.

Sen, R. & Broadhurst, K. 2011. Contact between children in out-of-home placements and their family and friends networks: A research review. *Child & Family Social Work*, 16(3), 298–309.

Shepherd, C., Reynolds, F. & Moran, J. 2010. "They're battle scars, I wear them well": A phenomenological exploration of young women's experiences of building resilience following adversity in adolescence. *Journal of Youth Studies*, 13(3), 273–290.

Shulman, J. 2014. *The Constitutional Parent: Rights, Responsibilities, and the Enfranchisement of the Child*. New Haven, CT: Yale University Press.

Simmonds, S. 2016. *Children in Custody 2015–16 An Analysis of 12–18-year-olds' Perceptions of Their Experiences in Secure Training Centres and Young Offender Institutions*. London: HM Inspectorate of Prisons/Youth Justice Board.

Simmons, R., Burgeson, R., Carlton, S. & Blyth, D. 1987. The Impact of Cumulative Change in Early Adolescence. *Child Development*, 58(5), 1220–1234.

Sinclair, I., Baker, C., Lee, J. & Gibbs, I. 2007. *The Pursuit of Permanence: A Study of the English Care System*. London: Jessica Kingsley Publishers.

Sinclair, I., Baker, C., Wilson, K., & Gibbs, I. 2005. *Foster Children: Where They Go and How They Get On*. London: Jessica Kingsley Publishers.

Sinclair, I., Parry, E., Biehal, N., Fresen, J., Kay, C., Scott, S. & Green, J. 2016. Multi-dimensional treatment foster care in England: Differential effects by level of initial antisocial behaviour. *European Child and Adolescent Psychiatry*, 25(8), 843–852.

Slade, E. & Wissow, L. 2007. The influence of childhood maltreatment on adolescents' academic performance. *Economics of Education Review,* 26, 604–614.

Sladović-Franz, B. & Branica, V. 2013. The relevance and experience of education from the perspective of Croatian youth in-care. *European Journal of Social Work,* 16(1), 137–152.

Smith, M. 2009. *Rethinking Residential Child Care: Positive perspectives.* Bristol: The Policy Press.

Smith, M. & Whyte, B. 2008. Social education and social pedagogy: Reclaiming a Scottish tradition in social work. *European Journal of Social Work,* 11(1), 15–28.

Social Exclusion Unit. 2003. *A Better Education for Children in Care.* London: Social Exclusion Unit (SEU)/Office of the Deputy Prime Minister.

Socialstyrelsen. 2011. *Barn och unga insatser 2010.* Stockholm: Socialstyrelsen.

Spratt, T., Nett, J., Bromfield, L., Hietamäki, J., Kindler, H. & Ponnert, L. 2015. Child protection in Europe: Development of an international cross-comparison model to inform national policies and practices. *British Journal of Social Work,* 45(5), 1508–1525.

Staines, J. 2016. *Risk, Adverse Influence and Criminalisation: Understanding the Over-Representation of Looked after Children in the Youth Justice System.* London: Prison Reform Trust/The Hadley Centre.

Stanley, N., Riordan, D. & Alaszewski, H. 2005. The mental health of looked-after children: Matching response to need. *Health and Social Care in the Community,* 13, 239–248.

Stein, M. 2006a. Research review: Young people leaving care. *Child & Family Social Work,* 11(2), 273–279.

Stein, M. 2006b. Young people aging out of care: The poverty of theory. *Children and Youth Services Review,* 28(4), 422–434.

Stein, M. 2008. Transitions from care to adulthood: Messages from research for policy and practice. In: Stein, M. & Munro, E. R. (eds). *Young People's Transitions from Care to Adulthood: International Research and Practice.* London: Jessica Kingsley Publishers, 289–307.

Stein, M. 2012. *Young People Leaving Care: Supporting Pathways to Adulthood.* London: Jessica Kingsley Publishers.

Stein, M. 2014. Young people's transitions from care to adulthood in European and Postcommunist Eastern European and Central Asian societies. *Australian Social Work,* 67(1), 24–38.

Stein, M. & Dumaret, A. 2011. The mental health of young people aging out of care and entering adulthood: Exploring the evidence from England and France. *Children and Youth Services Review,* 33(12), 2504–2511.

Stronach, E., Toth, S., Rogosch, F., Oshri, A., Todd Manly, J. & Cicchetti, D. 2011. Child maltreatment, attachment security, and internal representations of mother and mother–child relationships. *Child Maltreatment,* 16(2), 137–145.

Stone, S. 2007. Child maltreatment, out-of-home placement and academic vulnerability: A fifteen-year review of evidence and future directions. *Children and Youth Services Review,* 29(2), 139–161.

Stott, T. 2012. Placement instability and risky behaviors of youth aging out of foster care. *Child & Adolescent Social Work Journal,* 29(1), 61–83.

Stroufe, L. 2005. Attachment and development: A prospective, longitudinal study from birth to adulthood. *Attachment & Human Development,* 7(4), 349–367.

Sturgis, P. & Buscha, F. 2015. Increasing inter-generational social mobility: Is educational expansion the answer? *British Journal of Sociology,* 66(3), 512–533.

Sulimani-Aidan, Y. 2015. Do they get what they expect? The connection between young adults' future expectations before leaving care and outcomes after leaving care. *Children and Youth Services Review,* 55, 193–200.

Sung Hong, J., Algood, C., Chiu, Y.-L. & Lee, S. 2011. An ecological understanding of kinship foster care in the United States. *Journal of Child and Family Studies,* 20, 863–872.

Susman, E. & Rogol, A. 2004. Puberty and psychological development. In: Lerner, R. & Steinberg, L. *Handbook of Adolescent Psychology,* 2nd edition. Hoboken, NJ: John Wiley and Sons, Inc., 15–44.

Tan, J., Hessel, E., Loeb, E., Schad, M., Allen, J. & Chango, J. 2016. Long-Term Predictions From Early Adolescent Attachment State of Mind to Romantic Relationship Behaviors. *Journal of Research on Adolescence* 26(4), 1022–1035.

Tanaka, M., Wekerle, C., Schmuck, M. L., Paglia-Boak, A. 2011. The linkages among childhood maltreatment, adolescent mental health, and self-compassion in child welfare adolescents. *Child Abuse & Neglect* 35, 887–898.

The Care Inquiry. 2013. *Making not Breaking: Building Relationships for Our Most Vulnerable Children: Findings and Recommendations of the Care Inquiry.* London: The Care Inquiry.

Trede, W. 2008. Residential child care in European countries: Recent trends. In: Peters. F. (ed.) *Residential Child Care and Its Alternatives: International Perspectives.* Stoke on Trent: Trentham Books Limited, 21–31.

Trinder, L. 1996. Social work research: The state of the art (or science). *Child and Family Social Work,* 1, 233–242.

Trout, A., Hagaman, J., Casey, K., Reid, R. & Epstein, M. 2008. The academic status of children and youth in out-of-home care: A review of the literature. *Children and Youth Services Review,* 30(9), 979–994.

UCAS. 2016. *UCAS Undergraduate End of Cycle Reports 2016 End of Cycle Report.* Cheltenham: UCAS.

United Nations Committee on the Rights of the Child. 2009. *General Comment No. 12: The right of the child to be heard CRC/C/GC/12.* Geneva: United Nations.

United Nations Committee on the Rights of the Child. 2016a. *Concluding Observations on the Fifth Periodic Report of France CRC/C/FRA/CO/5.* Geneva: United Nations Office of the United Nations High Commissioner for Human Rights (OHCHR).

United Nations Committee on the Rights of the Child. 2016b. *Concluding Observations on the Combined Third and Fourth Periodic Reports of Ireland CRC/C/IRL/CO/3–4.* Geneva: Office of the United Nations High Commissioner for Human Rights (OHCHR).

United Nations Committee on the Rights of the Child. 2016c. *Concluding Observations on the Combined Third to Fifth Periodic Reports of Slovakia CRC/C/SVK/CO/3–5.* Geneva: Office of the United Nations High Commissioner for Human Rights (OHCHR).

United Nations Committee on the Rights of the Child. 2016d. *Concluding Observations on the fifth Periodic Report of the United Kingdom of Great Britain and Northern Ireland CRC/C/GBR/CO/5*. Geneva: Office of the United Nations High Commissioner for Human Rights (OHCHR).

United Nations Committee on the Rights of the Child. 2016e. *Concluding Observations on the Fifth Periodic Report of New Zealand CRC/C/NZL/CO/5*. Geneva: Office of the United Nations High Commissioner for Human Rights (OHCHR).

United Nations General Assembly (UNGA). 1989. *United Nations Convention on the Rights of the Child (UNCRC)*. Geneva: United Nations.

United Nations General Assembly (UNGA). 2010. *Guidelines for the Alternative Care of Children: Resolution/Adopted by the General Assembly, 24 February 2010, A/RES/64/142*, UNGA.

United States Interagency Council on Homelessness (USICH). 2013. *Framework to End Youth Homelessness: A Resource Text for Dialogue and Action*. Washington, DC: USICH.

Unrau, Y., Font, S. & Rawls, G. 2012. Readiness for college engagement among students who have aged out of foster care. *Children and Youth Services Review,* 34(1), 76–83.

U.S. Department of Health and Human Services, Administration for Children and Families, Administration on Children, Youth and Families, Children's Bureau. 2015. *Child Maltreatment 2013*. Washington, DC: U.S. Department of Health and Human Services.

Valdez, C., Lim, H. & Parker, C. 2015. Positive change following adversity and psychological adjustment over time in abused foster youth. *Child Abuse & Neglect,* 48, 80–91.

valentine, K. & Katz, I. 2015. How early is early intervention and who should get it? Contested meanings in determining thresholds for intervention. *Children and Youth Services Review,* 55, 121–127.

van den Dries, L., Juffer, F., van IJzendoorn, M. & Bakermans-Kranenburg, M. 2009. Fostering security? A meta-analysis of attachment in adopted children. *Children and Youth Services Review,* 31(3), 410–421.

van Eijck, F., Branje, S., Hale, W. & Meeus, W. 2012. Longitudinal associations between perceived parent-adolescent attachment relationship quality and generalized anxiety disorder symptoms in adolescence. *Journal of Abnormal Child Psychology,* 40, 871–883.

van Rooij, F., Maaskant, A., Weijers, I., Weijers, D. & Hermanns, J. 2015. Planned and unplanned terminations of foster care placements in the Netherlands: Relationships with characteristics of foster children and foster placements. *Children and Youth Services Review* 53, 130–136.

van Santen, E. 2015. Factors associated with placement breakdown initiated by foster parents – Empirical findings from Germany. *Child and Family Social Work,* 20(2), 191–201.

Vinnerljung, B. & Sallnäs, M. 2008. Into adulthood: A follow-up study of 718 young people who were placed in out-of-home care during their teens. *Child and Family Social Work,* 13(2), 144–155.

von Borczyskowski, A., Vinnerljung, B. & Hjern, A. 2013. Alcohol and drug abuse among young adults who grew up in substitute care – Findings from a Swedish national cohort study. *Children and Youth Services Review,* 35(12), 1954–1961.

von Stumm, S., Macintyre, S., Batty, D., Clark, H. & Deary, I. 2010. Intelligence, social class of origin, childhood behavior disturbance and education as predictors of status attainment in midlife in men: The Aberdeen Children of the 1950s study. *Intelligence,* 38, 202–211.

Wade, J., & Dixon, J. 2006. Making a home, finding a job: investigating early housing and employment outcomes for young people leaving care. *Child & Family Social Work*, 11(3), 199–208.

Wade, J. & Munro, E. 2008. UK. In: Stein, M. & Munro, E. (eds) *Young People's Transitions from Care to Adulthood: International Research and Practice.* London: Jessica Kingsley Publishers, 209–224.

Wade, J., Biehal, N., Farrelly, N. & Sinclair, I. 2010. *Maltreated Children in the Looked after System: A Comparison of Outcomes for Those Who Go Home and Those Who Do Not. DFE-RBX-10-06.* Department for Education.

Wade, J., Sinclair, I., Stuttard, L. & Simmonds, J. 2014. *Investigating Special Guardianship: Experiences, Challenges and Outcomes. Research Report DFE-RR372.* Department for Education.

Walsh, K., Fortier, M. & DiLillo, D. 2010. Adult coping with childhood sexual abuse: A theoretical and empirical review. *Agression and Violent Behavior,* 15, 1–13.

Weinberg, L., Oshiro, M. & Shea, N. 2014. Education liaisons work to improve educational outcomes of foster youth: A mixed methods case study. *Children and Youth Services Review,* 41, 45–52.

Welbourne, P. & Leeson, C. 2013. The education of children in care: A research review. In S. Jackson, *Pathways through Education for Young People in Care: Ideas from Research and Practice.* London: British Association for Adoption and Fostering (BAAF), 27–42.

White, K. 2008. Residential communities as a secure base. In: Peters, F. (ed.) *Residential Child Care and Its Alternatives: International Perspectives.* Stoke on Trent: Trentham Books Limited, 33–39.

Wigfall, V. & Cameron, C. 2006. Promoting young people's participation in research. In: Chase, E., Simon, A. & Jackson, S. *In Care and After: A Positive Perspective.* London: Routledge, 152–168.

Wilkins, D. 2012. Disorganised attachment indicates child maltreatment: How is this link useful for child protection social workers? *Journal of Social Work Practice,* 26(1), 15–30.

Williams, K., Papadopoulou, V. & Booth, N. 2012. *Prisoners' Childhood and Family Backgrounds: Results from the Surveying Prisoner Crime Reduction (SPCR) Longitudinal Cohort Study of Prisoners.* London: Ministry of Justice.

Winch, C. 2012. Vocational and civic education: Whither British policy? *Journal of Philosophy of Education,* 46(4), 603–618.

Winter, K. 2006. Widening our knowledge concerning young looked after children: The case for research using sociological models of childhood. *Child & Family Social Work,* 11(1), 55–64.

Wojciak, A., McWey, L. & Helfrich, C. 2013. Sibling relationships and internalizing symptoms of youth in foster care. *Children and Youth Services Review,* 35(7), 1071–1077.

Wolf, A. 2011. *Review of Vocational Education – The Wolf Report.* London: Department for Education.

Wolff, R., Biesel, K. & Heinitz, S. 2011. Child protection in an age of uncertainty: Germany's response. In: Gilbert, N., Parton, N. & Skivenes, M. (eds.). *Child Protection Systems: International Trends and Orientations.* New York: Oxford University Press, 183–203.

World Health Organisation. 2016. *International Statistical Classification of Diseases and Related Health Problems 10th Revision (ICD-10).* Available at: http://apps. who.int/classifications/icd10/browse/2016/en#/F90-F98 (Accessed 4 May 2016).

Wright, B., Barry, M., Hughes., E., Trépel, D., Ali, S. & Allgar, V. et al. 2015. Clinical effectiveness and cost-effectiveness of parenting interventions for children with severe attachment problems: A systematic review and meta-analysis. *Health Technol Assess,* 19(52), 1–347.

Yates, T., Byron Egeland, L. & Stroufe, A. 2003. Rethinking resilience. In S. Luthar (ed.). *Resilience and Vulnerability.* Cambridge: Cambridge University Press, 243–266.

Yu, P. & Delaney, J. 2016. The spread of higher education around the globe: A cross-country analysis of gross tertiary education enrollment, 1999–2005. *Educational Policy,* 30(2), 281–321.

Zeller, M. & Köngeter, S. 2012. Education in residential care and in school: A social-pedagogical perspective on the educational attainment of young women leaving care. *Children and Youth Services Review,* 34(6), 1190–1196.

Zetlin, A., Weinberg, L. & Shea, N. 2010. Caregivers, school liaisons, and agency advocates speak out about the educational needs of children and youths in foster care. *Social Work,* 55(3), 245–254.

Zolkoski, S. & Bullock, L. M. 2012. Resilience in children and youth: A review. *Children and Youth Services Review,* 34(12), 2295–2303.

Zorc, C., O'Reilly, A., Matone, M., Long, J., Watts, C. & Rubin, D. 2013. The relationship of placement experience to school absenteeism and changing schools in young, school-aged children in foster care. *Children and Youth Services Review,* 35(5), 826–833.

Index

admissions to schools 105
adolescence: attachment style
and disruption in 135–7, 159;
developmental tasks of 22–4; focal
model of 9, 10, 12, 13, 24–5, 56, 59,
80, 129, 137–9, 186–8; 'storm and
stress' theory of 24
adolescent agency 25
adolescent egocentrism 23
Adoption and Children Act 2002, 164
Adoption and Safe Families Act
1997, 17
adult advocate and educational
attainment of children 94
Adult Attachment Interview (AAI) 41
adulthood, transitioning to 22–8, 78
adult support and self-reliance of
children in care 147–9
African Americans and placement
instability 47
age: age of entry into care and
educational attainment 93; use of
coping strategies and 76
agency 25, 145, 146
agency neglect 159–63
aggression 36, 40
Allen, M. 88
Allik, J. 83
alternative care regimes 19–22; assessing
success of 21–2; social pedagogy in
20–1
Antisocial Process Screening
Device Callous-Unemotional
Scale 136
apprenticeship offer 87–8, 181
arenas of comfort 24–5, 138
Arnett, J. 23, 26, 85
aspirations of children in care 96–97
assets for autonomy 32–3

Association of Directors of Children's
Services (ADCS) 192
Atkins, L. 96
attachment 37–8; in childhood
impacting adult outcomes 40;
issues and maltreatment 12, 38–41;
placement stability and 45–7; resilient
adaptation and attachment styles 75;
state of mind 41; style in adolescence
and disruption 135–7, 159
attachment anxiety 40
attachment figure 37–9
attachment theory 9–10, 13, 37–41, 59,
129, 187
attainment gap *see* educational
attainment gap
Attention Deficit Hyperactivity Disorder
(ADHD) 36
autonomy 14, 29, 163, 189–90; full 28,
29, 31–3, 157, 189; interest of children
30; rights 10–11
avoidance coping strategy 76
avoidant attachment 40

Ball, S. 88
Bankston, C. 83
behavioural problems 37, 102;
attachment issues and 38–41
Bender, K. 5
bereavement in children's lives 41–5
Berlin, M. 84
Berridge, D. 116, 156
betrayal trauma theory 101
Biehal, N. 45, 186
Billett, S. 85
birth family: parents supporting
educational attainment 97;
relationships 137–9, 186; stress of 147
Boddy, J. 175